Dennis A. Smith,
Han van de Waterbeemd,
and Don K. Walker

**Pharmacokinetics and
Metabolism in Drug Design**

Methods and Principles in Medicinal Chemistry
Edited by R. Mannhold, H. Kubinyi, G. Folkers

Editorial Board
H.-D. Höltje, H. Timmerman, J. Vacca, H. van de Waterbeemd, T. Wieland

Previous Volumes of this Series:

Th. Dingermann, D. Steinhilber,
G. Folkers (eds.)

Molecular Biology in Medicinal Chemistry

Vol. 21

2004, ISBN 3-527-30431-2

H. Kubinyi, G. Müller (ed.)

Chemogenomics in Drug Discovery

Vol. 22

2004, ISBN 3-527-30987-X

T. I. Oprea (ed.)

Chemoinformatics in Drug Discovery

Vol. 23

2005, ISBN 3-527-30753-2

R. Seifert, T. Wieland (eds.)

G-Protein Coupled Receptors as Drug Targets

Vol. 24

2005, ISBN 3-527-30819-9

O. Kappe, A. Stadler

Microwaves in Organic and Medicinal Chemistry

Vol. 25

2005, ISBN 3-527-31210-2

W. Bannwarth, B. Hinzen (eds.)

Combinatorial Chemistry

Vol. 26, 2nd Ed.

2006, ISBN 3-527-30693-5

G. Cruciani (ed.)

Molecular Interaction Fields

Vol. 27

2005, ISBN 3-527-31087-8

M. Hamacher, K. Marcus, K. Stühler,
A. van Hall, B. Warscheid, H. E. Meyer
(eds.)

Proteomics in Drug Design

Vol. 28

2005, ISBN 3-527-31226-9

D. J. Triggle, M. Gopalakrishnan,
D. Rampe, W. Zheng (eds.)

Voltage-Gated Ion Channels as Drug Targets

Vol. 29

2006, ISBN 3-527-31258-7

D. Rognan

Ligand Design for G Protein-coupled Receptors

Vol. 30

2006, ISBN 3-527-31284-6

Dennis A. Smith, Han van de Waterbeemd,
and Don K. Walker

Pharmacokinetics and Metabolism in Drug Design

Second Revised Edition

WILEY-VCH Verlag GmbH & Co. KGaA

Series Editors

Prof. Dr. Raimund Mannhold
Molecular Drug Research Group
Heinrich-Heine-Universität
Universitätsstrasse 1
40225 Düsseldorf
Germany
Raimund.mannhold@uni-duesseldorf.de

Prof. Dr. Hugo Kubinyi
Donnersbergstrasse 9
67256 Weisenheim am Sand
Germany
kubinyi@t-online.de

Prof. Dr. Gerd Folkers
Collegium Helveticum
STW/ETH Zentrum
8092 Zürich
Switzerland
folkers@collegium.ethz.ch

Authors

Dr. Dennis A. Smith
Pfizer Global Research and Development
Sandwich Laboratories
Department of Drug Metabolism
Sandwich, Kent CT13 9NJ
UK
dennis.a.smith@pfizer.com

Dr. Han van de Waterbeemd
AstraZeneca
Alderley Park, Macclesfield
Cheshire SK10 4TG
UK
Han.VanDeWaterbeemd@astrazeneca.com

Dr. Don K. Walker
Pfizer Global Research and Development
Sandwich Laboratories
Department of Drug Metabolism
Sandwich, Kent CT13 9NJ
UK
don.walker@pfizer.com

Library of Congress Card No.: applied for
British Library Cataloguing-in-Publication Data
A catalogue record for this book is available from the British Library.

Bibliographic information published by Die Deutsche Bibliothek
Die Deutsche Bibliothek lists this publication in the Deutsche Nationalbibliografie; detailed bibliographic data is available in the Internet at <http://dnb.ddb.de>.

© 2006 WILEY-VCH Verlag GmbH & Co. KGaA, Weinheim

Printed in the Federal Republic of Germany
Printed on acid-free paper

Typesetting Kühn & Weyh, Satz und Medien, Freiburg
Printing betz-druck GmbH, Darmstadt
Bookbinding Litges & Dopf Buchbinderei GmbH, Heppenheim

ISBN-13: 978-3-527-31368-6
ISBN-10: 3-527-31368-0

Contents

Pharmacokinetics and Metabolism in Drug Design.
Dennis A. Smith, Han van de Waterbeemd, Don K. Walker (Eds.)
Copyright © 2006 WILEY-VCH Verlag GmbH & Co. KGaA, Weinheim
ISBN: 3-527-31368-0

A Personal Foreword to the First Edition

The concept of this book is simple. It represents the distillation of my experiences over 25 years within drug discovery and drug development, and in particular how the science of drug metabolism and pharmacokinetics impacts medicinal chemistry. Hopefully it will be a source of some knowledge, but more importantly, a stimulus for medicinal chemists wanting to understand as much as possible about the chemicals they make. As the work grew I realised it was impossible to fulfil the concept of this book without involving others. I am extremely grateful to my co-authors Don Walker and Han van de Waterbeemd for helping turn a skeleton into a fully clothed body, and in the process, contributing a large number of new ideas and directions. Upon completion of the book I realise how little we know and how much there is to do. Medicinal chemists often refer to the *magic methyl*. This term covers the small synthetic addition, which almost magically solves a discovery problem of transforming a mere ligand into a potential drug, beyond the scope of existing structure–activity relationships. A single methyl can disrupt crystal lattices, break hydration spheres, modulate metabolism, enhance chemical stability, displace water in a binding site and turns the sometimes weary predicable plod of methyl, ethyl, propyl, futile into methyl, ethyl, another methyl magic! This book has no magical secrets unfortunately, but time and time again the logical search for solutions is eventually rewarded by unexpected gains.

January 2001,   *Sandwich*
                                                                       Dennis A. Smith

Pharmacokinetics and Metabolism in Drug Design.
Dennis A. Smith, Han van de Waterbeemd, Don K. Walker (Eds.)
Copyright © 2006 WILEY-VCH Verlag GmbH & Co. KGaA, Weinheim
ISBN: 3-527-31368-0

A Personal Foreword to the Second Edition

I took great personal satisfaction in seeing our thoughts turned into a book, and sat back to relax. Very soon as I glanced at the book I saw gaps, missing links, things I wish we had said better or included. Pride turned gradually to frustration and provided the catalysis for a second edition. The experience spans 29 years, but my wonder and admiration for the magic of medicinal chemistry and those that practice it remain undimmed.

July 2005   *Dennis A. Smith*

Pharmacokinetics and Metabolism in Drug Design.
Dennis A. Smith, Han van de Waterbeemd, Don K. Walker (Eds.)
Copyright © 2006 WILEY-VCH Verlag GmbH & Co. KGaA, Weinheim
ISBN: 3-527-31368-0

Abbreviations and Symbols

Chapter 1

Abbreviations

CPC	Centrifugal partition chromatography
CoMFA	Comparative field analysis
3D-QSAR	Three-dimensional quantitative structure–activity relationships
HDM	Hexadecane membrane
IUPAC	International Union of Pure and Applied Chemistry
MLP	Molecular lipophilicity potential
RP-HPLC	Reversed-phase high-performance liquid chromatography
PAMPA	Parallel artificial membrane permeability assay
PGDP	Propylene glycol dipelargonate
PSA	Polar surface area
SF	Shake flask, referring to traditional method to measure $\log P$ or $\log D$
TPSA	Topological polar surface area

Symbols

AP_{SUV}	Absorption potential measured in small unilamellar vesicles (SUV)
$\Delta \log D$	Difference between $\log D$ in octanol/water and $\log D$ in alkane/water
$\Delta \log P$	Difference between $\log P$ in octanol/water and $\log P$ in alkane/water
f	Rekker or Leo/Hansch fragmental constant for $\log P$ contribution
K_a	Ionisation constant
Λ	Polarity term, mainly related to hydrogen bonding capability of a solute
$\log P$	Logarithm of the partition coefficient (P) of neutral species
$\log D$	Logarithm of the distribution coefficient (D) at a selected pH, usually assumed to be measured in octanol/water

Pharmacokinetics and Metabolism in Drug Design.
Dennis A. Smith, Han van de Waterbeemd, Don K. Walker (Eds.)
Copyright © 2006 WILEY-VCH Verlag GmbH & Co. KGaA, Weinheim
ISBN: 3-527-31368-0

$\log D_{oct}$	Logarithm of the distribution coefficient (D) at a selected pH, measured in octanol/water
$\log D_{chex}$	Logarithm of the distribution coefficient (D) at a selected pH, measured in cyclohexane/water
$\log D_{7.4}$	Logarithm of the distribution coefficient (D) at pH 7.4
MW	Molecular weight
π	Hansch constant; contribution of a substituent to log P
pK_a	Negative logarithm of the ionisation constant K_a

Chapter 2

Abbreviations

ADME	Absorption, distribution, metabolism and excretion
AUC	Area under plasma concentration time curve
CNS	Central nervous system
CYP2D6	Cytochrome P450 2D6 enzyme
GIT	Gastrointestinal tract
IV	Intravenous
PET	Positive emission tomography

Symbols

A_{av}	Average amount of drug in the body over a dosing interval
A_{max}	Maximum amount of drug in the body over a dosing interval
A_{min}	Minimum amount of drug in the body over a dosing interval
C_o	Initial concentration after IV dose
Cav_{ss}	Average plasma concentration at steady state
$C_{p(f)}$	Free (unbound) plasma concentration
$C_{p(fo)}$	Initial free (unbound) plasma concentration
C_{ss}	Steady state concentration
Cl	Clearance
Cl_u	Unbound clearance
Cl_H	Hepatic clearance
Cl_i	Intrinsic clearance
Cl_{iu}	Intrinsic clearance of unbound drug
Cl_o	Oral clearance
Cl_p	Plasma clearance
Cl_R	Renal clearance
Cl_S	Systemic clearance
D	Dose
E	Extraction
E_F	Fractional response
E_M	Maximum response
F	Fraction of dose reaching systemic circulation (bioavailability)
F_{da}	Fraction dose absorbed

f_u	Fraction of drug unbound
K_A	Affinity constant
K_B	Dissociation constant for a competitive antagonist
K_d	Dissociation constant
k_{el}	Elimination rate constant
K_m	Affinity constant (concentration at 50% V_{max})
k_o	Infusion rate
k_{+1}	Receptor on rate
k_{-1}	Receptor off rate
L	Ligand
$\log D_{7.4}$	Distribution coefficient (octanol/buffer) at pH 7.4
ln 2	Natural logarithm of two (i.e. 0.693)
pA_2	Affinity of antagonist for a receptor ($= -\log_{10}[K_B]$)
Q	Blood flow
R	Receptor
RL	Receptor ligand complex
RO	Receptor occupancy
s	Substrate concentration
t	Time after drug administration
T	Dosing interval
$t_{1/2}$	Elimination half-life
V_d	Volume of distribution
$V_{d(f)}$	Apparent volume of distribution of free (unbound) drug
V_{max}	Maximum rate of reaction (Michaelis–Menten enzyme kinetics)
ε	Dosing interval in terms of half-life ($= T / t_{1/2}$)

Chapter 3

Abbreviations

AUC	Area under plasma concentration time curve
Caco-2	Human colon adenocarcinoma cell line used as absorption model
GI	Gastrointestinal
MDCK	Madin–Darby canine kidney cell line used as absorption model
PSA	Polar surface area

Symbols

A%	Percentage of dose absorbed as measured in portal vein
CLOGP	MedChem/Biobyte log P estimation program
F%	Percentage of dose bioavailable
F_a	Fraction absorbed
F_{non}	Fraction non-ionised at pH of 6.5
IFV	Intestinal fluid volume (250 mL)
k_a	Absorption rate constant in rats (min^{-1})
log D	Logarithm of distribution coefficient

log P	Logarithm of partition coefficient
log S	Logarithm of solubility in water
RT	Average residence time in the small intestine (270 min)
$S_{6.5}$	Solubility in phosphate buffer at pH of 6.5
S_o	Intrinsic solubility of the neutral species at 37 °C
V_L	Volume of the lumenal contents
X_o	Dose administered

Chapter 4

Abbreviations

CNS	Central nervous system
CSF	Cerebrospinal fluid

Symbols

Cl_p	Plasma clearance
Cl_u	Unbound clearance of free drug
Δlog P	Difference in log P values in octanol and cyclohexane
H-bond	Hydrogen bond
k_{el}	Elimination rate constant
log $D_{7.4}$	Distribution coefficient at pH 7.4 (usually octanol/water)
log P	Partition coefficient (usually octanol)
pK_a	Ionisation constant
T_{max}	Time to maximum observed plasma concentration
$V_{d(f)}$	Unbound volume of distribution of the free drug

Chapter 5

Abbreviations

ATP	Adenosine triphosphate
BTL	Bilitranslocase
CYP450	Cytochrome P450
MOAT	Multiple organic acid transporter
MRP	Multi-drug resistance protein
Natp	Sodium dependent acid transporter protein
OATP	Organic acid transport protein
OCT1	Organic cation transporter 1
OCT2	Organic cation transporter 2
P-gp	P-glycoprotein
TxRA	Thromboxane receptor antagonist
TxSI	Thromboxane synthase inhibitor

Symbols

Cl	Clearance
$\log D_{7.4}$	Distribution coefficient (octanol/buffer) at pH 7.4
$t_{1/2}$	Elimination half-life
V_d	Volume of distribution

Chapter 6

Abbreviations

GFR	Glomerular filtration rate

Symbols

$C_{p(f)}$	Free (unbound) plasma concentration
$\log D_{7.4}$	Logarithm of distribution coefficient (octanol/buffer) at pH 7.4

Chapter 7

Abbreviations

COMT	Catechol-O-methyl transferase
CYP	Cytochrome P450
CYP2D6	2D6 isoenzyme of the cytochrome P450 enzyme family
CYP2C9	2C9 isoenzyme of the cytochrome P450 enzyme family
CYP3A4	3A4 isoenzyme of the cytochrome P450 enzyme family
FMO	Flavin mono-oxygenase
GST	Glutathione S-transferase
MAO	Monoamine oxidase
NEP	Neutral endopeptidase
P450	Cytochrome P450
PAPS	3'-Phosphoadenosine-5-phosphosulfate
UGT	UDP-glucuronosyltransferases

Symbols

$\log D_{7.4}$	Logarithm of the octanol/water distribution coefficient at pH 7.4
K_m	Affinity constant (concentration at 50% V_{max})

Chapter 8

Abbreviations

ANF	Atrial natriuretic factor (also ANP: atrial natriuretic peptide)
COX	Cyclooxygenase
ENCC	Electroneutral Na-Cl cotransporter
hFGF	Human fibroblast growth factor

GSH   Glutathione
HMG-CoA   3-Hydroxy-3-methylglutaryl coenzyme A
LH   Luteinizing hormone
5-LPO   5-Lipoxygenase
NK   Neurokinin
NKCC   Old name for ENCC
PBPK/PD   Physiologically-based pharmacokinetic/pharmacodynamic
             (modelling)
PCNA   Proliferating cell nuclear antigen
PPAR-γ Peroxisome proliferator-activated receptor γ
TA2   Thromboxane
VEGF   Vascular endothelial growth factor

Chapter 9

Abbreviations
BW Body weight
CYP2C9   Cytochrome P450 2C9 enzyme
GFR Glomerular filtration rate
IV   Intravenous
MLP   Maximum life span potential
P450   Cytochrome P450
TxRAs   Thromboxane receptor antagonists

Symbols
C_{max} Maximum plasma concentration observed
Cl Clearance
Cl_i Intrinsic clearance
Cl_{iu} Intrinsic clearance of unbound (free) drug
Cl_{ou} Oral unbound clearance (i.e. oral clearance correct for free fraction)
Cl_s Systemic clearance
f_b Fraction of plasma bound drug
f_u Fraction of drug unbound (to plasma proteins)
f_{ut} Fraction of unbound drug in tissues
ln   Natural logarithm
Q Organ blood flow
R Ratio of binding proteins in extracellular fluid (except plasma) to
             binding proteins in plasma
r^2 Correlation coefficient
$t_{1/2}$ Elimination half-life
V_d Volume of distribution
V_e Volume of extracellular fluid
V_p Volume of plasma
V_r Volume of remaining fluid

Chapter 10

Abbreviations

ADME	Absorption, distribution, metabolism, excretion
CYP3A4	Cytochrome P450 3A4
DMPK	Drug metabolism and pharmacokinetics
HTS	High-throughput screening
IAM	Immobilised artificial membrane
LC/MS	Liquid chromatography/mass spectrometry
MDR1	Gene coding for P-glycoprotein (P-gp); newer coding as ABCB1
MTS	Medium throughput screening
NADPH	Nicotinamide adenine dinucleotide phosphate
NMR	Nuclear magnetic resonance
PAMPA	Parallel artificial membrane permeability assay
PBPK	Physiologically-based pharmacokinetics
P-gp	P-glycoprotein
PK	Pharmacokinetics
PK/PD	Pharmacokinetics/pharmacodynamics
PSA	Polar surface area
QSAR	Quantitative structure–activity relationships
SAR	Structure–activity relationship
7TMs	Seven transmembrane loop receptors
UHTS	Ultra-high-throughput screening

Symbols

$\Delta \log P$	Difference between octanol/water and alkane/water $\log P$ as a measure for hydrogen bonding capacity
K_i	Binding constant (to receptor or metabolising enzyme)
$\log D_{7.4}$	Logarithm of the octanol/water distribution coefficient at pH 7.4
$\log P$	Logarithm of the octanol/water partition coefficient for the neutral species
$\log S_w$	Logarithm of the aqueous solubility
MW	Molecular weight

1
Physicochemistry

1.1
Physicochemistry and Pharmacokinetics

The body can be viewed as primarily composed of a series of membrane barriers dividing aqueous filled compartments. These membrane barriers are comprised principally of the phospholipid bilayers, which surround cells and also form intracellular barriers around the organelles present in cells (mitochondria, nucleus, etc.). These are formed with the polar ionised head groups of the phospholipid facing towards the aqueous phases and the lipid chains providing a highly hydrophobic inner core. To cross the hydrophobic inner core a molecule must also be hydrophobic and able to shed its hydration sphere. Many of the processes of drug disposition depend on the ability or inability to cross membranes and hence there is a high correlation with measures of lipophilicity. Moreover, many of the proteins involved in drug disposition have hydrophobic binding sites further adding to the importance of the measures of lipophilicity [1].

At this point it is appropriate to define the terms hydrophobicity and lipophilicity. According to recently published IUPAC recommendations both terms are best described as follows [2]:

- Hydrophobicity is the association of non-polar groups or molecules in an aqueous environment, which arises from the tendency of water to exclude non-polar molecules.
- Lipophilicity represents the affinity of a molecule or a moiety for a lipophilic environment. It is commonly measured by its distribution behaviour in a biphasic system, either liquid–liquid (e.g. partition coefficient in 1-octanol/water) or solid–liquid (retention on reversed-phase high-performance liquid chromatography (RP-HPLC) or thin-layer chromatography (TLC) system).

Further key physicochemical properties include solubility/dissolution and the ionisation state [3]. All these properties have a strong influence on absorption [4], membrane permeability, volume of distribution and to a certain extent metabolism [5]. The role of dissolution in the absorption process is also discussed under Section 3.2. Other properties closely linked to the physicochemical behaviour of

Pharmacokinetics and Metabolism in Drug Design.
Dennis A. Smith, Han van de Waterbeemd, Don K. Walker (Eds.)
Copyright © 2006 WILEY-VCH Verlag GmbH & Co. KGaA, Weinheim
ISBN: 3-527-31368-0

molecules are the structural features molecular weight and hydrogen-bonding capacity, which can be seen as the main contributors to log P/D.

1.2
Partition and Distribution Coefficient as Measures of Lipophilicity

The inner hydrophobic core of a membrane can be modelled by the use of an organic solvent. Similarly a water or aqueous buffer can be used to mimic the aqueous filled compartment. If the organic solvent is not miscible with water then a two phase system can be used to study the relative preference of a compound for the aqueous (hydrophilic) or organic (hydrophobic, lipophilic) phase.

For an organic compound, lipophilicity can be described in terms of its partition coefficient P (or log P as it is generally expressed). This is defined as the ratio of concentrations of the compound at equilibrium between the organic and aqueous phases:

$$P = \frac{[\text{drug}]_{\text{organic}}}{[\text{drug}]_{\text{aqueous}}} \tag{1.1}$$

The partition coefficient (log P) describes the *intrinsic lipophilicity* of the collection of functional groups and carbon skeleton, which combine, to make up the structure of the compound, *in the absence of dissociation or ionisation*. Methods to measure partition and distribution coefficients have been described [6, 7].

Every component of an organic compound has a defined lipophilicity and calculation of partition coefficient can be performed from a designated structure. Likewise, the effect on log P of the introduction of a substituent group into a compound can be predicted by a number of methods as pioneered by Hansch (π values) [8–11], Rekker (f values) [12, 13], and Leo and Hansch (f' values) [8–10, 14, 15].

Partitioning of a compound between aqueous and lipid (organic) phases is an equilibrium process. When in addition, the compound is partly ionised in the aqueous phase a further (ionisation) equilibrium is set up, since it is assumed that under normal conditions only the unionised form of the drug penetrates the organic phase [16]. This traditional view is shown schematically in Fig. 1.1 below. However, the nature of the substituents surrounding the charged atom as well as the degree of delocalisation of the charge may contribute to the stabilisation of the ionic species and thus not fully exclude partitioning into an organic phase or membrane [17]. An example of this is the design of acidic 4-hydroxyquinolones (Fig. 1.2) as glycine/NMDA antagonists [18]. Despite a formal negative charge these compounds appear to be have considerable blood-brain barrier crossing.

In a study of the permeability of alfentanil and cimetidine through Caco-2 cells (Fig. 1.3), a model for oral absorption, it was deduced that at pH 5 ca. 60% of the cimetidine transport and 17% of the alfentanil transport across Caco-2 monolayers can be attributed to the ionised form [19]. Thus the dogma that only neutral species can cross a membrane has been challenged recently.

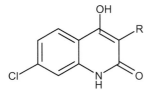

1. Is a function of acid/base strength pK_a
2. Is a function of P (log P)

Fig. 1.1 Schematic depicting the relationship between log P and log D and pK_a.

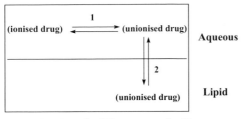

Fig. 1.2 4-Hydroxyquinolines with improved oral absorption and blood-brain barrier permeability [18].

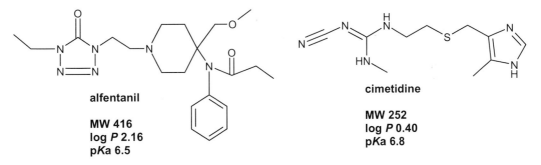

alfentanil

MW 416
log P 2.16
pKa 6.5

cimetidine

MW 252
log P 0.40
pKa 6.8

Fig. 1.3 Rapidly (alfentanil) and slowly (cimetidine) trans ported basic drugs across Caco-2 monolayers [19].

The intrinsic lipophilicity (P) of a compound refers only to the equilibrium of the unionised drug between the aqueous phase and the organic phase. It follows that the remaining part of the overall equilibrium, i.e. the concentration of ionised drug in the aqueous phase, is also of great importance in the overall observed partition ratio. This in turn depends on the pH of the aqueous phase and the acidity or basicity (pK_a) of the charged function. The overall ratio of drug, ionised and unionised, between the phases has been described as the *distribution coefficient* (D), to distinguish it from the intrinsic lipophilicity (P). The term has become widely used in recent years to describe, in a single term the *effective* (or *net*) *lipophilicity* of a compound at a given pH taking into account both its intrinsic lipophilicity and its degree of ionisation. The distribution coefficient (D) for a monoprotic acid (HA) is defined as:

$$D = [HA]_{organic} / ([HA]_{aqueous} + [A^-]_{aqueous}) \tag{1.2}$$

where [HA] and [A$^-$] represent the concentrations of the acid in its unionised and dissociated (ionised) states, respectively. The ionisation of the compound in water is defined by its dissociation constant (K_a) as:

$$K_a = [H^+][A^-] / [HA] \tag{1.3}$$

sometimes referred to as the Henderson–Hasselbalch relationship. Combination of Eqs. 1.1–1.3 gives the pH distribution relationship:

$$D = P / (1 + \{K_a / [H^+]\}) \tag{1.4}$$

more commonly expressed for monoprotic organic acids in the form of Eqs. 1.5 and 1.6, below:

$$\log (\{P / D\} - 1) = pH - pK_a \tag{1.5}$$

or

$$\log D = \log P - \log (1 + 10^{pKa - pH}) \tag{1.6}$$

For monoprotic organic bases (BH$^+$ dissociating to B) the corresponding relationships are:

$$\log (\{P / D\} - 1) = pK_a - pH \tag{1.7}$$

or

$$\log D = \log P - \log (1 + 10^{pH - pKa}) \tag{1.8}$$

From these equations it is possible to predict the effective lipophilicity (log D) of an acidic or basic compound at any pH value. The data required in order to use the relationship in this way are the intrinsic lipophilicity (log P), the dissociation constant (pK_a), and the pH of the aqueous phase. The overall effect of these relationships is that the effective lipophilicity of a compound, at physiological pH; is the log P value minus one unit of lipophilicity, for every unit of pH the pK_a value is below (for acids) and above (for bases) pH of 7.4. Obviously for compounds with multifunctional ionisable groups the relationship between log P and log D, as well as log D as functions of pH become more complex [20]. For diprotic molecules there are already twelve different possible shapes of log D – pH plots.

1.3
Limitations on the Use of 1-Octanol

Octanol is the most widely used model of a biological membrane [21, 22] and log $D_{7.4}$ values above zero normally correlate with effective transfer across the lipid core of the membrane, whilst values below zero suggest an inability to traverse the hydrophobic barrier.

Octanol, however, supports H-bonding. Besides the free hydroxyl group, octanol also contains 4% v/v water at equilibrium. This obviously conflicts with the exclusion of water and H-bonding functionality at the inner hydrocarbon core of the membrane. Therefore, for compounds that contain functionality capable of forming H-bonds, the octanol value can over-represent the actual membrane crossing ability. These compounds can be thought of as having a high hydration potential and have difficulty in shedding their water sphere.

Use of a hydrocarbon solvent such as cyclohexane can discriminate these compounds either as the only measured value or as a value to be subtracted from the octanol value (Δlog P) [23–25]. Unfortunately, cyclohexane is a poor solvent for many compounds and does not have the utility of octanol. Groups which hydrogen bond and attenuate actual membrane crossing compared to their predicted ability based on octanol are listed in Fig. 1.4. The presence of two or more amide, carboxyl functions in a molecule will significantly impact membrane crossing ability and will need substantial intrinsic lipophilicity in other functions to provide sufficient hydrophobicity to penetrate the lipid core of the membrane.

Octanol/Cyclohexane Ratio (H-bonding) →

Alkyl Phenyl Halogen	Amine Ester Ether Ketone Nitrile Nitro	Sec Amide Amide *Pri* Amine Carboxylate Hydroxyl Sulfonamide Sulfone Sulfoxide

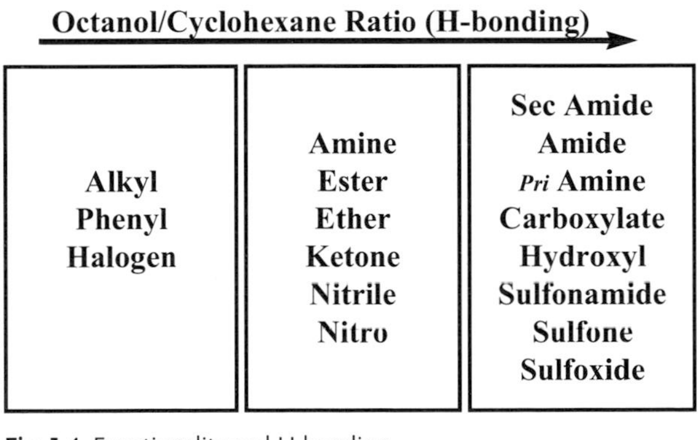

Fig. 1.4 Functionality and H-bonding.

1.4
Further Understanding of Log *P*

1.4.1
Unravelling the Principal Contributions to Log *P*

The concept that log *P* or log *D* is composed of two components [26], that of size and polarity is a useful one. This can be written as

$$\log P \text{ or } \log D = a \cdot V - \Lambda \tag{1.9}$$

where *V* is the molar volume of the compound, *Λ* a general polarity descriptor, and *a* is a regression coefficient. Thus the size component will largely reflect the carbon skeleton of the molecule (lipophilicity) whilst the polarity will reflect the hydrogen-bonding capacity. The positioning of these properties to the right and left in Fig. 1.4 reflects their influence on the overall physicochemical characteristics of a molecule.

1.4.2
Hydrogen Bonding

Hydrogen bonding is now seen as an important property related to membrane permeation. Various scales expressing H-bonding have been developed [27]. Some of these scales describe total hydrogen-bonding capability of a compound, while others discriminate between donors and acceptors [28]. It was demonstrated that most of these scales show considerable intercorrelation [29].

Lipophilicity and H-bonding are important parameters for uptake of drugs in the brain [30]. Their role has been studied in a series of structurally diverse, sedating and non-sedating, histamine H_1 receptor antagonists [31]. From these studies a decision tree guideline for the development of non-sedative anti-histamines was designed (see Fig. 1.5).

GABA (*γ*-aminobutyric acid) is a major neurotransmitter in mammals and is involved in various CNS (central nervous system) disorders. In the design of a series of GABA uptake inhibitors a large difference in *in vivo* activity between two compounds with identical IC_{50} values was observed, one compound being devoid of activity [32]. The compounds have also nearly identical pK_a and log D_{oct} values (see Fig. 1.6) and differ only in their distribution coefficient of cyclohexane/water (log D_{chex}). This results in a Δlog *D* of 2.71 for the *in vivo* inactive compounds, which is believed to be too large for CNS uptake. The active compound has a Δlog *D* of 1.42, well below the critical limit of around 2. Besides this physicochemical explanation, further evaluation of metabolic differences should complete this picture. It should be noted that the concept of using the differences between solvent systems was originally developed for compounds in their neutral state (Δlog *P* values, see Section 2.2). In this case two zwitterions are being compared, which are considered at pH of 7.4 to have a net zero charge, and thus the Δlog *P* concept seems applicable.

Considerable interest is focused on the calculation of hydrogen-bonding capability for use in quantitative structure–activity relationships (QSAR) studies, design of combinatorial libraries, and for correlation with absorption and permeability data [33–35]. A number of different descriptors for hydrogen bonding have been discussed [36], one of the simplest being the count of the number of hydrogen bond-forming atoms [37].

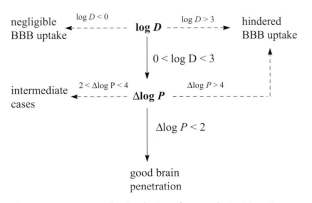

Fig. 1.5 Decision tree for the design of non-sedative H$_1$ antihistaminics. Log D is measured at pH 7.4, while Δlog P refers to compounds in their neutral state (redrawn from [31]).

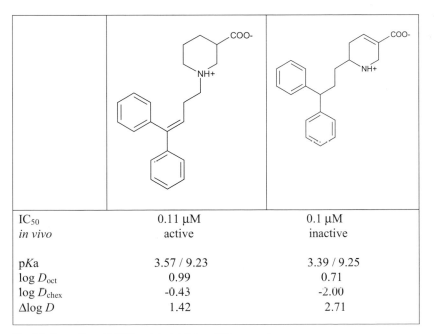

IC$_{50}$	0.11 μM	0.1 μM
in vivo	active	inactive
pKa	3.57 / 9.23	3.39 / 9.25
log D_{oct}	0.99	0.71
log D_{chex}	-0.43	-2.00
Δlog D	1.42	2.71

Fig. 1.6 Properties of GABA-uptake inhibitors [32].

A simple measure of hydrogen-bonding capacity is polar surface area (*PSA*), summing up the fractional contributions to surface area of all nitrogen and oxygen atoms [38]. This was used to predict passage of the blood-brain barrier [39, 40], flux across a Caco-2 monolayer [41], and human intestinal absorption [42, 43]. The physical explanation is that polar groups are involved in desolvation when they move from an aqueous extracellular environment to the more lipophilic interior of membranes. *PSA* thus represents, at least part, of the energy involved in membrane transport. *PSA* is dependent on the conformation and the original method is based on a single minimum energy conformation [38]. Others have taken into account conformational flexibility and coined a dynamic *PSA*, in which a Boltzmann-weighted average *PSA* is computed [42]. However, it was demonstrated that the *PSA* calculated for a single minimum energy conformation is in most cases sufficient to produce a sigmoidal relationship to intestinal absorption (see Fig 3.12), differing very little from the dynamic *PSA* described above [43]. A fast calculation of *PSA* as a sum of fragment-based contributions, called topological polar surface area (*TPSA*), has been published [44], allowing the use of these calculations for large data sets such as combinatorial or virtual libraries. The sigmoidal relationship can be described by $A\% = 100 \, / \, [1 + (PSA \, / \, PSA_{50})^{\gamma}]$, where $A\%$ is the percentage of orally absorbed drug, PSA_{50} is the *PSA* at 50% absorption level, and γ is a regression coefficient. Others have used a Boltzmann sigmoidal curve given by $y = \text{bottom} + (\text{top} - \text{bottom}) \, / \, (1 + \exp[(x_{50} - x)/\text{slope}])$ [43].

Poorly absorbed compounds have been identified as those with a $PSA > 140 \, \text{Å}^2$. Considering more compounds, considerably more scatter was found around the sigmoidal curve observed for a smaller set of compounds [43]. This is partly due to the fact that many compounds do not show simple passive diffusion only, but are affected by active carriers, efflux mechanisms involving P-glycoprotein (P-gp) and other transporter proteins, and gut wall metabolism. A further refinement in the *PSA* approach is expected to come from taking into account the strength of the hydrogen bonds, which in principle is the basis of the hydrogen bond thermodynamics approach.

1.4.3
Molecular Size and Shape

Molecular size can be a limiting factor in oral absorption. The Lipinski *rule of five* proposes an upper limit of (molecular weight) *MW* 500 as acceptable for orally absorbed compounds [45]. Molar volume as used in Eq. 1.9 is another way to express the size of a compound. It is very much related to molecular surface area. For convenience often the molecular weight is taken as a first estimate of size. It is also useful to realise that size is not identical to shape. Size and shape parameters are generally not measured, but rather calculated. A measured property is the so-called cross-sectional area, which is obtained from surface activity measurements [46].

Molecular weight is often taken as the size descriptor of choice, while it is easy to calculate and is in the chemist's mind. However, other size and shape properties are equally as simple to calculate and may offer a better guide to estimate the potential for permeability. Thus far no systematic work has been reported investigating this in detail. Cross-sectional area A_D obtained from surface activity measurements have been reported as a useful size descriptor to discriminate between compounds, which can access the brain ($A_D < 80\,\text{Å}^2$) of those that are too large to cross the blood-brain barrier [46]. Similar studies have been performed to define a cut-off for oral absorption [47].

Many companies have tried to develop peptidic renin inhibitors. Unfortunately these are rather large molecules and not unexpectedly poor absorption was often observed. The role of physicochemical properties has been discussed for this class of compounds. One of the conclusions was that compounds with higher lipophilicity were better absorbed in the intestine [48]. Absorption and bile elimination rate both are *MW*-dependent. Lower *MW* gives better absorption and less bile excretion. The combined influence of molecular size and lipophilicity on absorption of a series of renin inhibitors can be seen in Fig. 1.7. The observed isosize curves are believed to be part of a general sigmoidal relationship between permeability and lipophilicity [49–51] (see Chapter 3).

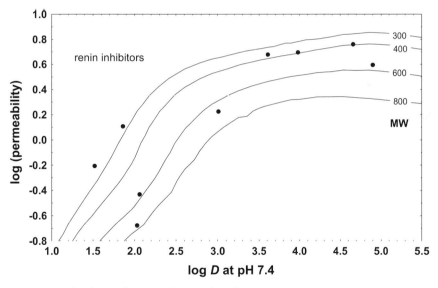

Fig. 1.7 Isomolecular weight curves showing the influence of molecular size on membrane permeability with increasing lipophilicity [51].

1.5
Alternative Lipophilicity Scales

1.5.1
Different Solvent Systems

Since 1-octanol has certain limitations (see Section 1.3) many alternative lipophilicity scales have been proposed [52] (see Fig. 1.3). A critical quartet of four solvent systems of octanol (amphiprotic), alkane (inert), chloroform (proton donor) and propylene glycol dipelargonate (PGDP) has been advocated [53, 54]. By measuring distribution in all four a full coverage of partitioning properties should have been obtained. Also non-aqueous systems such as heptane/acetonitrile [55] or heptane/glycol [56] may be of use. This latter system appears to offer a direct measure for hydrogen bonding. Alkane/water partitioning is thought to be a good imitation of the blood-brain barrier. Hexadecane/water partitioning and distribution can be measured in a PAMPA-like set-up using hexadecane membranes (HDM) [57] (for PAMPA see Chapter 3).

1.5.2
Chromatographic Approaches

In order to increase throughput over the traditional shake flask and related methods, various chromatographic techniques can be used [1]. Particularly, immobilised artificial membranes (IAM) had considerable attention [58, 59]. IAMs consist of phospholipids grafted on a solid phase HPLC support intended to mimic membrane character (see Fig. 1.8). It appears that IAM retention times are highly correlated with shake flask log D octanol/water coefficients and thus do not really measure something different.

1.5.3
Liposome Partitioning

Several groups have suggested that studying partitioning into liposomes may produce relevant information related to membrane uptake and absorption [59, 60]. Liposomes, which are lipid bilayer vesicles prepared from mixtures of lipids, provide a useful tool for studying passive permeability of molecules through lipids. This system has been used to demonstrate the passive nature of the absorption mechanism of monocarboxylic acids [61]. Liposome partitioning of ionisable drugs can be determined by titration and has been correlated with human absorption [62]. A new absorption potential parameter has been suggested, as calculated from liposome distribution data and the solubility-dose ratio, which shows an excellent sigmoidal relationship with human passive intestinal absorption (Eq. 1.10) [62–64].

$$AP_{SUV} = \log \left(\text{Distribution} \times \text{Solubility} \times V / \text{Dose} \right) \qquad (1.10)$$

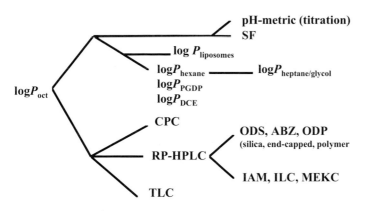

Fig. 1.8 Experimental methods to measure lipophilicity (modified after [26]). Key of abbreviations-log P_{oct}:1-octanol/water partition coefficient, log $P_{liposomes}$: partition coefficient between liposomes and buffer, log P_{hexane}: 1-hexane/water partition coefficient, log P_{PGDP}: propyleneglycol dipelargonate/water partition coefficient, log $P_{heptane/glycol}$: a non-aqueous partitioning system, SF: shake flask, pH-metric: log P determination based on potentiometric titration in water and octanol/water, CPC: centrifugal partition chromatography, RP-HPLC: reversed-phase high-performance liquid chromatography, TLC: thin-layer chromatography, ODS: octadecylsilane, ABZ: end-capped silica RP-18 column, ODP: octadecylpolyvinyl packing, IAM: immobilised artificial membrane, ILC: immobilised liposome chromatography, MEKC: micellar electrokinetic capillary chromatography.

Here, AP_{SUV} is the absorption potential measured from the distribution in small unilamellar vesicles (SUV) at pH 6.8, the solubility was measured at pH 6.8 in simulated intestinal fluid, V is the volume of intestinal fluid, and dose is a mean single oral dose. Liposome partitioning is only partly correlated with octanol/water distribution.

A further partition system based on the use of liposomes, and commercialised under the name Transil, has been investigated [52, 65, 66].

1.6
Computational Approaches to Lipophilicity

In the design of new compounds as well as the design of experimental procedures an a priori calculation log P or log D values may be very useful. Methods may be based on the summation of fragmental [67–69], or atomic contributions [70–72], or a combination [73, 74]. Reviews of various methods can be found in Refs. [67, 75–78]. Further approaches based on the use of structural features have been suggested [75, 79]. Atomic and fragmental methods suffer from the problem that not all contributions may be parameterised. This leads to the observation that for a typical pharmaceutical file ca. 25% of the compounds cannot be computed. Recent efforts try to improve the *missing value* problem [80].

Molecular lipophilicity potential (MLP) has been developed as a tool in 3D-QSAR, for the visualisation of lipophilicity distribution on a molecular surface and as an additional field in CoMFA studies [76]. MLP can also be used to estimate conformation-dependent log *P* values.

1.7
Membrane Systems to Study Drug Behaviour

In order to overcome the limitations of octanol, other solvent systems have been suggested. Rather than a simple organic solvent, actual membrane systems have also been utilised. For instance the distribution of molecules has been studied between unilamellar vesicles of dimyristoylphosphatidylcholine and aqueous buffers. These systems allow the interaction of molecules to be studied with the whole membrane, which includes the charged polar head group area (hydrated)

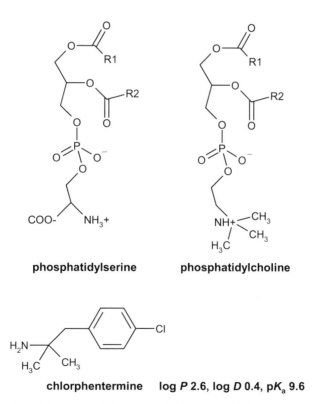

phosphatidylserine   **phosphatidylcholine**

chlorphentermine   **log *P* 2.6, log *D* 0.4, p*K*ₐ 9.6**

Fig. 1.9 Structures of charge neutral (phosphatidylcholine) and acidic (phosphatidylserine) phospholipids together with the moderately lipophilic and basic drug chlorphentermine. The groupings R1 and R2 refer to the acyl chains of the lipid portions.

and the highly lipophilic carbon chain region. Such studies indicate that partitioning for amine compounds ionised at physiological pH, partitioning into the membrane is highly favoured and independent of the degree of ionisation. This is believed to be due to electrostatic interactions with the charged phospholipid head group. This property is not shared with acidic compounds even for the *electronically neutral* phosphatidylcholine [81]. Such ionic interactions between basic drugs are even more favoured for membranes containing *acidic* phospholipids such as phosphatidylserine [82]. The structures of these two phospholipids are shown in Fig. 1.9, together with the structure of the basic drug chlorphentermine.

Table 1.1 shows the preferential binding of chlorphentermine for phosphatidylcholine-containing membranes, the phospholipid with overall acidic charge. These systems predict actually affinity for the membrane, rather than the ability to transfer across a membrane. Membrane affinity, and hence tissue affinity, is particularly important in the persistence of drugs within the body. This topic will be covered under volume of distribution in Chapter 4.

Tab. 1.1 Affinity (*k*) and capacity (moles drug/moles lipid) of chlorphentermine for liposomes prepared from phosphatidylcholine and phosphatidylserine.

Phospholipid	*k* [10^{-4}] M	n_{max}
Phosphatidylserine	2.17	0.67
Phosphatidylcholine	1.26	0.05

1.8
Dissolution and Solubility

1.8.1
Why Measure Solubility?

Each cellular membrane can be considered as a combination of a physicochemical and biological barrier to drug transport. Poor physicochemical properties may sometimes be overcome by an active transport mechanism. Before any absorption can take place at all, the first important properties to consider are dissolution and solubility. Many cases of solubility-limited absorption have been reported and therefore solubility is now seen as a property to be addressed at early stages of drug discovery. Only a compound in solution is available for permeation across the gastrointestinal membrane. Solubility has long been recognised as a limiting factor in the absorption process leading to the implementation of solubility screens in early stages of drug design [45, 83]. High-throughput solubility measurements have been developed, which can be used in early discovery [45, 84–86].

Excessive lipophilicity is a common cause of poor solubility and can lead to erratic and incomplete absorption following oral administration. Estimates of desired solubility for good oral absorption depend on the permeability of the compound and the required dose, as illustrated in Table 1.2 [83].

Tab. 1.2 Desired solubility correlated to expected doses [83].

Dose (mg kg^{-1})	Permeability		
	High	Medium	Low
0.1	1*	5	21
1	10	52	207
10	100	520	2100

* $\mu g\ mL^{-1}$

The incorporation of an ionisable centre, such as an amine or similar function, into a template can bring a number of benefits including water solubility (see Chapter 3).

Dissolution testing has been used as a prognostic tool for oral drug absorption [87]. A biopharmaceutical classification scheme (BCS) has been proposed, under which drugs can be categorised into four groups according to their solubility and permeability properties [88]. Because both permeability as well as solubility can be further dissected into more fundamental properties, it has been argued that the principal properties are not solubility and permeability, but rather molecular size and hydrogen bonding [89]. The BCS has been adopted as a regulatory guidance for bioequivalence studies.

1.8.2
Calculated Solubility

As a key first step towards oral absorption, considerable effort went into the development of computational solubility prediction [90–94]. However, partly due to a lack of large sets of experimental data measured under identical conditions, today's methods are not robust enough for reliable predictions [95]. Further fine-tuning of the models can be expected now as high-throughput data becomes available to construct such models.

1.9
Ionisation (pK_a)

Drug ionisation has an important effect in the *in vitro* prediction of *in vivo* absorption [96]. Various ways an ion may cross a membrane have been described [97]. These include transport as ion (trans- and/or para-cellular), ion pair, or protein-assisted (using the outer surface of a protein spanning a membrane).

The dogma based on the pH-partition theory that only neutral species cross a membrane has been challenged [98]. An example was already discussed above for studies with Caco-2 monolayers that suggested that the ionic species may contribute considerably to overall drug transport [18]. Using cyclic voltammetry it was also demonstrated that compounds in their ionised form pass into organic phases and might well cross membranes in this ionised form [99].

Therefore a continued interest exists in the role of pK_a in absorption, which often is related to its effect on lipophilicity and solubility. New methods to measure pK_a values are being explored, e.g. using electrophoresis, and an instrument for high-throughput pK_a measurement has been developed [100].

The difference between the log P of a given compound in its neutral form (log P^N) and its fully ionised form (log P^I) has been termed *diff*(log P^{N-I}) and contains series-specific information, and expresses the influence of ionisation on the intermolecular forces and intramolecular interactions of a solute [99]. It is unclear at present how these latter concepts can be used in drug design.

References

1 Pliska, V., Testa, B., Van de Waterbeemd, H. (eds.) **1996**, *Lipophilicity in Drug Action and Toxicology*, VCH, Weinheim.

2 a) Van de Waterbeemd, H., Carter, R.E., Grassy, G., Kubinyi, H., Martin, Y.C., Tute, M.S., Willett, P. **1997**, *Pure Chem.* 69, 1137–1152. b) Van de Waterbeemd, H., Carter, R.E., Grassy, G., Kubinyi, H., Martin, Y.C., Tute, M.S., Willett, P. **1998**, *Ann. Rep. Med. Chem.* 33, 397–409.

3 Van de Waterbeemd, H. **2002**, Physicochemical properties, in *Medicinal Chemistry: Principles and Practice*, King, F.D. (ed.), 2nd edn, RSC, London.

4 Van de Waterbeemd, H., Lennernas, H., Artursson, P. **2003**, *Drug Bioavailability*, Wiley-VCH, Weinheim.

5 Van de Waterbeemd, H., Smith, D.A., Beaumont, K., Walker, D.K. **2001**, *J. Med. Chem.* 44, 1313–1333.

6 Dearden, J.C., Bresnen, G.M. **1988**, *Quant. Struct. Act. Relat.* 7, 133–144.

7 Hersey, A., Hill, A.P., Hyde, R.M., Livingstone, D.J. **1989**, *Quant. Struct. Act. Relat.* 8, 288–296.

8 Hansch, C., Leo, A. **1979**, *Substituent Constants for Correlation Analysis in Chemistry and Biology*, Wiley-Interscience, New York.

9 Hansch, C., Leo, A., Hoekman, D. **1995**, *Exploring QSAR: Hydrophobic, Electronic, and Steric Constants*, ACS, Washington, D.C.

10 Hansch, C., Leo, A. **1995**, *Exploring QSAR: Fundamentals and Applications in Chemistry and Biology*, ACS, Washington, D.C.

11 Fujita, T., Iwasa, J., Hansch, C. **1964**, *J. Amer. Chem. Soc.* 86, 5175–5180.

12 Rekker, R.F., De Kort, H.M. **1979**, *Eur. J. Med. Chem.* 14, 479–488.

13 Rekker, R.F., Mannhold, R. **1992**, *Calculation of Drug Lipophilicity*, VCH, Weinheim.

14 Leo, A., Abraham, D.J. **1988**, *Proteins: Struct. Funct. Gen.* 2, 130–152.

15 Leo, A., Hansch, C., Elkins, D. **1971**, *Chem. Revs* 71, 525–616.

16 Manners, C.N., Payling, D.W., Smith, D.A. **1988**, *Xenobiotica* 18, 331–350.

17 Kulagowski, J.J., Baker, R., Curtis, N.R., Leeson, P.D., Mawer, I.M., Moseley, A.M., Ridgill, M.P., Rowley, M., Stansfield, I., Foster, A.C., Gromwood, S., Hill, R.G., Kemp, J.A., Marshall, G.R., Saywell, K.L., Tricklebank, M.D. **1994**, *J. Med. Chem.* 37, 1402–1405.

18 Palm, K., Luthman, K., Ros, J., Grasjo, J., Artursson, P. **1999**, *J. Pharmacol. Exp. Ther.* 291, 435–443.

19 Reymond, F., Carrupt, P.A., Testa, B., Girault, H.H. **1999**, *Chem. Eur. J.* 5, 39–47.

20 Smith, R.N., Hansch, C., Ames, M.M. **1975**, *J. Pharm. Sci.* 64, 599–605.

21 Avdeef, A. **1996**, Assessment of distribution-pH profiles, in *Lipophilicity in Drug Action and Toxicology*, Pliska, V., Testa, B., Van de Waterbeemd, H. (eds.), VCH, Weinheim, (pp.) 109–139.

22 Avdeef, A. **2003**, *Absorption and Drug Development*, Wiley-Interscience, Hoboken, NJ.

23 Young, R.C., Mitchell, R.C., Brown, T.H., Ganellin, C.R., Griffiths, R., Jones, M., Rana, K.K., Saunders, D., Smith, I.R., Sore, N.E., Wilks, T.J. **1998**, *J. Med. Chem.* 31, 656–671.

24 El Tayar, N., Tsai, R.S., Testa, B., Carrupt, P.A., Leo, A. **1991**, *J. Pharm. Sci.* 80, 590–598.

25 Abraham, M.H., Chadha, H.S., Whiting, G.S., Mitchell, R.C. **1994**, *J. Pharm. Sci.* 83, 1085–1100.

26 Van de Waterbeemd, H., Testa, B. **1987**, *Adv. Drug Res.* 16, 85–225.

27 Van de Waterbeemd, H. **2000**, Intestinal permeability: prediction from theory, in *Methods for Assessing Oral Drug Absorption*, Dressman, J. (ed.), Dekker, New York, (pp.) 31–49.

28 Abraham, M.H., Chadra, H.S., Martins, F., Mitchell, R.C. **1999**, *Pestic. Sci.* 55, 78–99.

29 Van de Waterbeemd, H., Camenisch, G., Folkers, G., Raevsky, O.A. **1996**, *Quant. Struct. Act. Relat.* 15, 480–490.

30 Van de Waterbeemd, H., Camenisch, G., Folkers, G., Chretien, J.R., Raevsky, O.A. **1998**, *J. Drug Target* 6, 151–165.

31 Ter Laak, A.M., Tsai, R.S., Donné-Op den Kelder, G.M., Carrupt, P.A., Testa, B. **1994**, *Eur. J. Pharm. Sci.* 2, 373–384.

32 N'Goka, V., Schlewer, G., Linget, J.M., Chambon, J.-P., Wermuth, C.-G. **1991**, *J. Med. Chem.* 34, 2547–2557.

33 Raevsky, O.A., Schaper, K.-J. **1998**, *Eur. J. Med. Chem.* 33, 799–807.

34 Raevsky, O.A., Fetisov, V.I., Trepalina, E.P., McFarland, J.W., Schaper, K.-J. **2000**, *Quant. Struct. Act. Relat.* 19, 366–374.

35 Van de Waterbeemd, H., Camenisch, G., Folkers, G., Raevsky, O.A. **1996**, *Quant. Struct. Act. Relat.* 15, 480–490.

36 Van de Waterbeemd, H. **2000**, Intestinal permeability: prediction from theory, in *Oral Drug Absorption*, Dressman, J.B., Lennernas, H. (eds.), Dekker, New York, (pp.) 31–49.

37 Österberg, T., Norinder, U. **2000**, *J. Chem. Inf. Comput. Sci.* 40, 1408–1411.

38 Van de Waterbeemd, H., Kansy, M. **1992**, *Chimia* 46, 299–303.

39 Kelder, J., Grootenhuis, P.D.J., Bayada, D.M., Delbressine, L.P.C., Ploemen, J.-P. **1999**, *Pharm. Res.* 16, 1514–1519.

40 Clark, D.E. **1999**, *J. Pharm. Sci.* 88, 815–821.

41 Camenisch, G., Folkers, G., Van de Waterbeemd, H. **1997**, *Int. J. Pharmaceut.* 147, 61–70.

42 Palm, K., Luthman, K., Ungell, A.-L., Strandlund, G., Beigi, F., Lundahl, P., Artursson, P. **1998**, *J. Med. Chem.* 41, 5382–5392.

43 Clark, D.E. **1999**, *J. Pharm. Sci.* 88, 807–814.

44 Ertl, P., Rohde, B., Selzer, P. **2000**, *J. Med. Chem.* 43, 3714–3717.

45 Lipinski, C.A., Lombardo, F., Dominy, B.W., Feeney, P.J. **1997**, *Adv. Drug. Del. Revs.* 23, 3–25.

46 Fischer, H., Gottschlich, R., Seelig, A. **1998**, *J. Membr. Biol.* 165, 201–211.

47 Fischer, H. **1998**, Dissertation, University of Basel, Switzerland.

48 Hamilton, H.W., Steinbaugh, B.A., Stewart, B.H., Chan, O.H., Schmid, H.L., Schroeder, R., Ryan, M.J., Keiser, J., Taylor, M.D., Blankley, C.J., Kaltenbronn, J.S., Wright, J., Hicks, J. **1995**, *J. Med. Chem.* 38, 1446–1455.

49 Camenisch, G., Folkers, G., Van de Waterbeemd, H. **1996**, *Pharm. Acta. Helv.* 71, 309–327.

50 Camenisch, G., Folkers, G., Van de Waterbeemd, H. **1998**, *Eur. J. Pharm. Sci.* 6, 321–329.

51 Van de Waterbeemd, H. **1997**, *Eur. J. Pharm. Sci. Suppl.* 2, S26–S27.

52 Hartmann, T., Schmitt, J. **2004**, *Drug Disc. Today: Technol.* 1, 431–439.

53 Leahy, D.E., Taylor, P.J., Wait, A.R. **1989**, *Quant. Struct. Act. Relat.* 8, 17–31.

54 Leahy, D.E., Morris, J.J., Taylor, P.J., Wait, A.R. **1992**, *J. Chem. Soc. Perkin. Trans.* 2, 723–731.

55 Suzuki, N., Yoshida, Y., Watarai, H. **1982**, *Bull. Chem. Soc. Jpn.* 55, 121–125.

56 Paterson, D.A., Conradi, R.A., Hilgers, A.R., Vidmar, T.J., Burton, P.S. **1994**, *Quant. Struct. Act. Relat.* 13, 4–10.

57 Wohnsland, F., Faller, B. **2001**, *J. Med. Chem.* 44, 923–930.

58 Yang, C.Y., Cai, S.J., Liu, H., Pidgeon, C. **1996**, *Adv. Drug Del. Revs.* 23, 229–256.

59 Ottiger, C., Wunderli-Allenspach, H. **1999**, *Pharm. Res.* 16, 643–650.

60 Balon, K., Riebesehl, B.U., Muller, B.W. **1999**, *Pharm. Res.* 16, 882–888.

61 Takagi, M., Taki, Y., Sakane, T., Nadai, T., Sezaki, H., Oku, N., Yamashita, S. **1998**, *J. Pharmacol. Exp. Ther.* 285, 1175–1180.

62 Balon, K., Riebesehl, B.U., Muller, B.W. **1999**, *Pharm. Res.* 16, 882–888.

63 Balon, K., Riebesehl, B.U., Muller, B.W. **1999**, *J. Pharm. Sci.* 88, 802–806.

64 Avdeef, A., Box, K.J., Comer, J.E.A., Hibbert, C., Tam, K.Y. **1998**, *Pharm. Res.* 15, 209–215.

65 Escher, B.I., Schwarzenbach, R.P., Westall, J.C. **2000**, *Environ. Sci. Technol.* 34, 3962–3968.

66 Loidl-Stahlhofen, A., Eckrt, A., Hartmann, T., Schottner, M. **2001**, *J. Pharm. Sci.* 90, 599–606.

67 Leo, A. **1993**, *Chem. Revs.* 93, 1281–1308.

68 Mannhold, R., Rekker, R.F., Dross, K., Bijloo, G., De Vries, G. **1998**, *Quant. Struct. Act. Relat.* 17, 517–536.

69 Rekker, R.F., Mannhold, R., Bijloo, G., De Vries, G., Dross, K. **1998**, *Quant. Struct. Act. Relat.* 17, 537–548.

70 Kellogg, G.E., Joshi, G.S., Abraham, D.J. **1992**, *Med. Chem. Res.* 1, 444–453.

71 Viswanadhan, V.N., Ghose, A.K., Revankar, G.R., Robins, R.K. **1989**, *J. Chem. Inf. Comput. Sci.* 29, 163–172.

72 Ghose, A.K., Crippen, G.M. **1987**, *J. Chem. Inf. Comput. Sci.* 27, 21–35.

73 Meylan, W.M., Howard, P.H. **1995**, *J. Pharm. Soc.* 84, 83–92.

74 Spessard, G.O. **1998**, *J. Chem. Inf. Comput. Sci.* 38, 55–57.

75 Buchwald, P., Bodor, N. **1998**, *Curr. Med. Chem.* 5, 353–380.

76 Carrupt, P.A., Testa, B., Gaillard, P. **1997**, *Revs. Comput. Chem.* 11, 241–315.

77 Van de Waterbeemd, H., Mannhold, R. **1996**, *Quant. Struct. Act. Relat.* 15, 410–412.

78 Mannhold, R., Van de Waterbeemd, H. **2002**, *J. Comput. Aided. Mol. Des.* 15, 337–354.

79 Moriguchi, I., Hirono, S., Nakagome, I., Hirano, H. **1994**, *Chem. Pharm. Bull.* 42, 976–978.

80 Leo, A.J., Hoekman, D. **2000**, *Perspect. Drug Disc. Des.* 18, 19–38.

81 Austin, R.P., Davis, A.M., Manners, C.N. **1995**, *J. Pharm. Sci.* 84, 1180–1183.

82 Lullman, H., Wehling, M. **1979**, *Biochem. Pharmacol.* 28, 3409–3415.

83 Lipinski, C. **2000**, *J. Pharm. Tox. Meth.* 44, 235–249.

84 Bevan, C.D., Lloyd, R.S. **2000**, *Anal. Chem.* 72, 1781–1787.

85 Avdeef, A. **2001**, High-throughput measurements of solubility profiles, in *Pharmacokinetic Optimization in Drug Research; Biological, Physicochemical and Computational Strategies*, Testa, B., Van de Waterbeemd, H., Folkers, G., Guy, R. (eds.) Wiley-VCH, Weinheim, (pp.) 305–325.

86 Avdeef, A., Berger, C.M. **2001**, pH-Metric solubility 3, *Eur. J. Pharm. Sci.* 14, 281–291.

87 Dressman, J.B., Amidon, G.L.,
Reppas, C., Shah, V.P. **1998**, *Pharm.
Res.* 15, 11–22.

88 Amidon, G.L., Lennernäs, H.,
Shah, V.P., Crison, J.R.A. **1995**,
Pharm. Res. 12, 413–420.

89 Van de Waterbeemd, H. **1998**, *Eur. J.
Pharm. Sci.* 7, 1–3.

90 Huuskonen, J. **2001**, *Comb. Chem.
High Throughput Scr.* 4, 311–316.

91 McFarland, J.W., Avdeef, A., Berger,
C.M., Raevsky, O.A. **2001**, *J. Chem. Inf.
Comput. Sci.* 41, 1355–1359.

92 Livingstone, D.J., Ford, M.G., Huuskonen, J.J., Salt, D.W. **2001**, *J. Comput.
Aid. Mol. Des.* 15, 741–752.

93 Bruneau, P. **2001**, *J. Chem. Inf. Comput.
Sci.* 41, 1605–1616.

94 Liu, R., So, S.-S. **2001**, *J. Chem. Inf.
Comput. Sci.* 4, 1633–1639.

95 Van de Waterbeemd, H. **2002**, *Curr.
Opin. Drug Disc. Dev.* 5, 33–43.

96 Boisset, M., Botham, R.P., Haegele,
K.D., Lenfant, B., Pachot, J.L. **2000**, *Eur.
J. Pharm. Sci.* 10, 215–224.

97 Camenisch, G., Van de Waterbeemd,
H., Folkers, G. **1996**, *Pharm. Acta. Helv.*
71, 309–327.

98 Pagliara, A., Resist, M., Geinoz, S.,
Carrupt, P.-A., Testa, B. **1999**, *J. Pharm.
Pharmacol.* 51, 1339–1357.

99 Caron, G., Gaillard, P., Carrupt, P.A.,
Testa, B. **1997**, *Helv. Chim. Acta* 80,
449–461.

100 Kerns, E.H., Di, L. **2004**, *Drug Disc.
Today: Technol.* 1, 343–348.

2
Pharmacokinetics

2.1
Setting the Scene

Pharmacokinetics is the study of the time course of a drug within the body and incorporates the processes of absorption, distribution, metabolism and excretion (ADME). In general, pharmacokinetic parameters are derived from the measurement of drug concentrations in blood or plasma. The simplest pharmacokinetic concept is that based on the total drug in plasma. However, drug molecules may be bound at a greater or lesser extent to the proteins present within the plasma, thus free drug levels may be vastly different from those of the total drug. Blood or plasma are the traditionally sampled matrices due to (a) convenience and (b) that the concentrations in the circulation will be in some form of equilibrium with the tissues of the body. Because of analytical difficulties (separation, sensitivity) it is usually the total drug that is measured and used in pharmacokinetic evaluation. Such measurements and analysis are adequate for understanding a single drug in a single species in a number of different situations since protein binding and resultant unbound fraction is approximately constant under these conditions. When species or drugs are compared, certain difficulties arise in the use of total drug and the unbound (free) drug is a more useful measure (see Section 2.9).

2.2
Intravenous Administration: Volume of Distribution

When a drug is administered intravenously into the circulation the compound undergoes distribution into tissues etc., and clearance. For a drug that undergoes rapid distribution a simple model can explain the three important pharmacokinetic terms: volume of distribution, clearance and half-life.

Volume of distribution (V_d) is a theoretical concept that connects the administered dose with the actual initial concentration (C_0) present in the circulation. The relationship is shown below.

$$V_d = \text{Dose} / C_0 \qquad (2.1)$$

Pharmacokinetics and Metabolism in Drug Design.
Dennis A. Smith, Han van de Waterbeemd, Don K. Walker (Eds.)
Copyright © 2006 WILEY-VCH Verlag GmbH & Co. KGaA, Weinheim
ISBN: 3-527-31368-0

For a drug that is confined solely to the circulation (blood volume is 80 mL kg^{-1}), the volume of distribution will be 0.08 L kg^{-1}. Distribution into total body water (800 mL kg^{-1}) results in a volume of distribution of 0.8 L kg^{-1}. Beyond these values the number has only a mathematical importance. For instance a volume of distribution of 2 L kg^{-1} means only that less than 5% of the drug is present in the circulation. The drug may be generally distributed to many tissues and organs or concentrated in only a few.

For different molecules, the apparent volume of distribution may range from about 0.04 L kg^{-1} to more than 20 L kg^{-1}. High molecular weight dyes, such as indocyanine green, are restricted to the circulating plasma after intravenous administration and thus exhibit a volume of distribution of about 0.04 L kg^{-1}. For this reason such compounds are used to estimate plasma volume and hepatic blood flow [1, 2]. Certain ions, such as chloride and bromide, rapidly distribute throughout extracellular fluid, but do not readily cross cell membranes and therefore exhibit a volume of distribution of about 0.4 L kg^{-1} which is equivalent to the extracellular water volume [3]. Neutral lipid soluble substances can distribute rapidly throughout intracellular and extracellular water. For this reason antipyrine has been used as a marker of total body water volume and exhibits a volume of distribution of about 0.7 L kg^{-1} [4]. Compounds which bind more favourably to tissue proteins than plasma proteins can exhibit apparent volumes of distribution far in excess of the body water volume. This is because the apparent volume is dependent on the ratio of free drug fractions in the plasma and tissue compartments [5]. High tissue affinity is most commonly observed with basic drugs and can lead to apparent volumes of distribution up to 21 L kg^{-1} for the primary amine containing calcium channel blocker, amlodipine [6].

2.3
Intravenous Administration: Clearance

Clearance of drug occurs by the perfusion of the blood to the organs of extraction. Extraction (E) refers to the proportion of drug presented to the organ that is removed irreversibly (excreted) or altered to a different chemical form (metabolism). Clearance (Cl) is therefore related to the flow of blood through the organ (Q) and is expressed by the formula:

$$Cl = Q \cdot E \tag{2.2}$$

The organs of extraction are generally the liver (hepatic clearance-metabolism and biliary excretion, Cl_H) and the kidney (renal excretion, Cl_R), and the values can be summed together to give an overall value for systemic clearance (Cl_S):

$$Cl_S = Cl_H + Cl_R \tag{2.3}$$

Extraction is the ratio of the clearance process compared to the overall disappearance of the compound from the organ. The clearance process is termed intrinsic clearance Cl_i, the other component of disappearance is the blood flow (Q) from the organ. This is shown in Fig. 2.1 below.

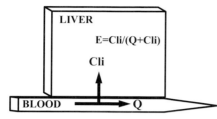

Fig. 2.1 Schematic illustrating hepatic extraction with Q, blood flow and Cl_i, intrinsic clearance (metabolism).

Combining Eq. 2.2 and Eq. 2.3 with the scheme in Fig. 2.1 gives the general equation for clearance of:

$$Cl = Q \cdot Cl_i / (Q + Cl_i) \tag{2.4}$$

Where $Cl = Cl_S$ if only one organ is involved in drug clearance. Within this equation Cl_i is the intrinsic clearance based on total drug concentrations and therefore includes drug bound to protein. Lipophilic drugs bind to the constituents of plasma (principally albumin) and in some cases to erythrocytes. It is a major assumption, supported by a considerable amount of experimental data, that only the unbound (free) drug can be cleared. The intrinsic clearance (Cl_i) can be further defined as:

$$Cl_i = Cl_{iu} \times f_u \tag{2.5}$$

Where Cl_{iu} is the intrinsic clearance of free drug, i.e. unrestricted by either flow or binding, and f_u is the fraction of drug unbound in blood or plasma.

Inspection of the above equation indicates for compounds with low intrinsic clearance compared to blood flow, Q and ($Cl_i + Q$) effectively cancel and Cl (or Cl_S) approximates to Cl_i. Conversely, when intrinsic clearance is high relative to blood flow, Cl_i and ($Cl_i + Q$) effectively cancel and Cl (or Cl_S) is equal to blood flow (Q). The implications of this on drugs cleared by metabolism is that the systemic clearance of low-clearance drugs are sensitive to changes in metabolism rate whereas that of high clearance drugs are sensitive to changes in blood flow.

It is important to recognise the distinction between the various terms used for drug clearance and the interrelationship between these. Essentially intrinsic clearance values are independent of flow through the organ of clearance, whilst unbound clearance terms are independent of binding. These relationships are illustrated in Fig. 2.2.

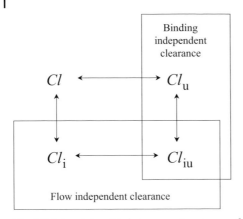

Fig. 2.2 Interrelationship between various terms of drug clearance used within pharmacokinetic analysis.

2.4
Intravenous Administration: Clearance and Half-life

Clearance is related to the concentrations present in blood after administration of a drug by the equation:

$$Cl = \text{Dose} / \text{AUC} \tag{2.6}$$

where AUC is the area under the plasma concentration time curve. Clearance is a constant with units often given as mL min^{-1} or mL per min per kg body weight. These values refer to the volume of blood totally cleared of drug per unit time. Hepatic blood flow values are 100, 50 and 25 mL per min per kg in rat, dog and man. Blood clearance values approaching these indicate that hepatic extraction is very high (rapid metabolism).

Blood arriving at an organ of extraction normally contains only a fraction of the total drug present in the body. The flow through the major extraction organs, the liver and kidneys, is about 3% of the total blood volume per minute; however, for many drugs, distribution out of the blood into the tissues will have occurred. The duration of the drug in the body is therefore the relationship between the clearance (blood flow through the organs of extraction and their extraction efficiency) and the amount of the dose of drug actually in the circulation (blood). The amount of drug in the circulation is related to the volume of distribution and so the elimination rate constant (k_{el}) is given by the relationship:

$$k_{el} = Cl / V_d \tag{2.7}$$

The elimination rate constant can be described as a proportional rate constant. An elimination rate constant of 0.1 hour^{-1} means that 10% of the drug is removed per hour.

The elimination rate constant and half-life $(t_{1/2})$, the time taken for the drug concentration present in the circulation to decline to 50% of the current value, are related by the equation:

$$t_{1/2} = \ln 2 \; / \; k_{el} \tag{2.8}$$

Half-life reflects how often a drug needs to be administered. To maintain concentrations with minimal peak and trough levels over a dosing interval, a rule of thumb is that the dosing interval should equal the drug half-life. Thus for once a day administration, a 24 hour half-life is required. This will provide a peak to trough variation in plasma concentration of approximately twofold. In practice the tolerance in peak to trough variation in plasma concentration will depend on the therapeutic index of a given drug and dosing intervals of two to three half-lives are not uncommon.

The importance of these equations is that drugs can have different half-lives due either to changes in clearance or changes in volume (see Section 2.7). This is illustrated in Fig. 2.3 for a simple single compartment pharmacokinetic model where half-life is doubled either by reducing clearance to 50% or doubling the volume of distribution.

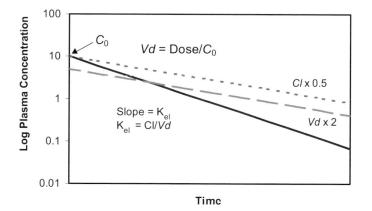

Fig. 2.3 Effect of clearance and volume of distribution on half-life for a simple single compartment pharmacokinetic model.

2.5
Intravenous Administration: Infusion

With linear kinetics, providing an intravenous infusion is maintained long enough, a situation will arise when the rate of drug infused equals the rate of drug eliminated. The plasma or blood concentrations will remain constant and be described as *steady state*. The plasma concentration profile following intravenous infusion is illustrated in Fig. 2.4.

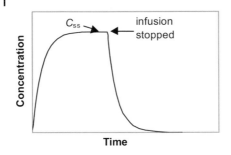

Fig. 2.4 Plasma concentration profile observed after intravenous infusion.

The steady state concentration (C_{ss}) is defined by the equation:

$$C_{ss} = k_o \,/\, Cl_p \qquad\qquad (2.9)$$

where k_o is the infusion rate and Cl_p is the plasma (or blood) clearance. The equation which governs the rise in plasma concentration is shown below where the plasma concentration (C_p) may be determined at any time (t).

$$C_p = k_o \,/\, Cl_p \,(1 - \exp[-k_{el} \cdot t]) \qquad\qquad (2.10)$$

Thus the time taken to reach steady state is dependant on k_{el}. The larger k_{el} (shorter the half-life) the more rapidly the drug will attain steady state. As a guide 87% of steady state is attained when a drug is infused for a period equal to three half-lives. Decline from steady state will be as described above, so a short half-life drug will rapidly attain steady state during infusion and rapidly disappear following the cessation of infusion.

Increasing the infusion rate will mean the concentrations will climb until a new steady state value is obtained. Thus doubling the infusion rate doubles the steady state plasma concentration as illustrated in Fig. 2.5.

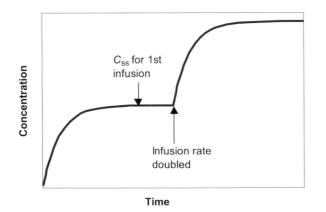

Fig. 2.5 Intravenous infusion with infusion rate doubled.

2.6
Oral Administration

When a drug is administered orally, the drug has to be absorbed across the membranes of the gastrointestinal tract. Incomplete absorption lowers the proportion of the dose able to reach the systemic circulation. The blood supply to the gastrointestinal tract (GIT) is drained via the hepatic portal vein, which passes through the liver on its passage back to the heart and lungs. Transport of the drug from the gastrointestinal tract to the systemic circulation will mean the entire absorbed dose has to pass through the liver (Fig. 2.6).

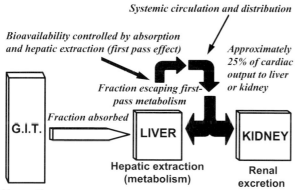

Fig. 2.6 Schematic illustrating the disposition of a drug after oral administration.

On this *first-pass* the entire dose is subjected to liver extraction and the fraction of the dose reaching the systemic circulation (*F*) can be substantially reduced (even for completely absorbed drugs) as shown in the following equation:

$$F = 1 - E \qquad (2.11)$$

Again E is the same concept as that shown in Fig. 2.1. This phenomenon is termed the first-pass effect, or pre-systemic metabolism, and is a major factor in reducing the bioavailability of lipophilic drugs. From the concept of extraction in Fig. 2.1, rapidly metabolised drugs, with high Cl_i values, will have high extraction and high first-pass effects. An example of this type of drug is the lipophilic, calcium channel blocker, felodipine. This compound has an hepatic extraction of about 0.80, leading to oral systemic drug exposure (based on AUC) only about one fifth of that observed after intravenous administration [7]. Conversely, slowly metabolised drugs, with low Cl_i values, will have low extraction and show small and insignificant first-pass effects. The class III anti-dysrhythmic drug, dofetilide, provides such an example. Hepatic extraction of this compound is only about 0.07, leading to similar systemic exposure (AUC) after oral and intravenous doses [8].

A complication of this can be additional first-pass effects caused by metabolism by the gastrointestinal tract itself. In the most extreme cases, such as midazolam, extraction by the gut wall may be as high as 0.38 to 0.54 and comparable to that of the liver itself [9].

The previous equations for intravenously administered drugs (e.g. Eq. 2.6) can be modified to apply to the oral situation:

$$Cl_o = F \cdot \text{Dose} / \text{AUC} \tag{2.12}$$

Where Cl_o is the oral clearance and F indicates the fraction absorbed and escaping hepatic first-pass effects. Referring back to the intravenous equation we can calculate F or absolute bioavailability by administering a drug intravenously and orally and measuring drug concentrations to derive the respective AUCs. When the same dose of drug is given then:

$$F = \text{AUC}_{\text{oral}} / \text{AUC}_{\text{IV}} \tag{2.13}$$

The estimation of systemic clearance together with this value gives valuable information about the behaviour of a drug. High clearance drugs with values approaching hepatic blood flow will indicate hepatic extraction (metabolism) as a reason for low bioavailability. In contrast poor absorption will probably be the problem in low-clearance drugs which show low bioavailabilities.

2.7
Repeated Doses

When oral doses are administered far apart in time they behave independently. This is usually not the desired profile if we assume that a certain concentration is needed to maintain efficacy, and if a certain concentration is exceeded, side effects will occur. Giving doses of the drug sufficiently close together so that the following doses are administered prior to the full elimination of the preceding dose means that some accumulation will occur. Moreover, a smoothing out of the plasma concentration profile will occur. This is illustrated in Fig. 2.7.

Ultimately if doses are given very close together then the effect is that of intravenous infusion and a steady state occurs. In fact for any drug an average steady state value (Cav_{ss}) can be calculated:

$$Cav_{ss} = F \cdot \text{Dose} / Cl \cdot T \tag{2.14}$$

where T is the interval between doses, dose is the size of the single administered dose and Cl is clearance. Note that $F \cdot \text{Dose} / T$ in this equation is actually the dosing rate as for intravenous infusion.

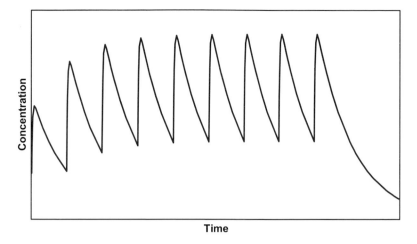

Fig. 2.7 Plasma concentration profile for multiple oral dose administration.

The same relationship to k_{el} and half-life also apply, so that as with intravenous infusion 87.5% of the final steady state concentration is achieved following administration of the drug for three half-lives.

This equation can be rewritten to indicate amount of drug in the body by substitution of k_{el} for Cl_o. Since k_{el} equals $0.693/t_{1/2}$, the equation below emerges:

$$A_{av} = 1.44 \cdot F \cdot t_{1/2} \cdot (\text{Dose} / T) \tag{2.15}$$

where A_{av} is the average amount of drug in the body over the dosing interval. By relating this to each dose an accumulation ratio (R_{ac}) can be calculated:

$$R_{ac} = A_{av} / F \cdot \text{Dose} = 1.44 \cdot t_{1/2} / T \tag{2.16}$$

The maximum and minimum amounts in the body (A_{max} and A_{min}, respectively) are defined by:

$$A_{max} = \text{Dose} / 1 - (1/2)^{\varepsilon} \tag{2.17}$$

$$A_{min} = \text{Dose} \cdot 1[1 - (1/2)^{\varepsilon} - 1] \tag{2.18}$$

where $\varepsilon = T / t_{1/2}$ or the dosing interval defined in terms of half-life. These equations mean that for a drug given once a day with a twenty-four hour half-life then a steady state will be largely achieved in three to four days. In addition, the amount of drug in the body (or the plasma concentration) will be approximately 1.4 times that of a single dose and that this will fluctuate between approximately twice the single dose and equivalent to the dose.

2.8
Development of the Unbound (Free) Drug Model

As outlined before, pharmacokinetics based on total drug concentrations proves useful in many situations, but is limited when data from a series of compounds are compared. This is the normal situation in a drug discovery programme and alternative presentations of pharmacokinetic information need to be explored. Since the medicinal chemist is trying to link compound potency in *in vitro* systems (receptor binding, etc.) with behaviour *in vivo*, it is important to find ways to unify the observations.

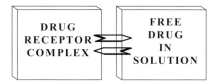

Fig. 2.8 Schematic illustrating equilibrium between drug and receptor.

Measurement of the unbound drug present in the circulation, and basing pharmacokinetic estimates on this, allows the *in vitro* and *in vivo* data to be rationalised.

The first and possibly the simplest biological test for a drug is the *in vitro* assessment of affinity for its target. Such experiments can be shown schematically as in Fig. 2.8 in which the drug is added to the aqueous buffer surrounding the receptor (or cell or tissue) and the total drug added is assumed to be in aqueous solution and in equilibrium with the receptor.

2.9
Unbound Drug and Drug Action

The biological or functional response to receptor activation can be assumed to be directly proportional to the number of receptors (R) occupied by a given ligand (L) at equilibrium. This assumption is termed the occupancy theory of drug response. The equation describing this phenomenon was proposed as:

$$[R] \; E_F / E_M = [RL] / [R]_T \tag{2.19}$$

where E_F is the fractional response, E_M is the maximal response, $[RL]$ is the concentration of receptor/ligand complex and $[R]_T$ is the total receptor concentration. At equilibrium, $R + L \Leftrightarrow RL$, such that the affinity constant K_A can be defined as $K_A = [RL] / [L][R]$. This is the same equation derived from Langmuir's saturation isotherm, which derives from the law of mass action. It is possible to describe the occupancy theory in the following way:

- The receptor/ligand (RL) complex is reversible.
- Association is a bimolecular process.
- Dissociation is a monomolecular process.
- All receptors of a given type are equivalent and behave independently from one another.
- The concentration of ligand is greatly in excess of the receptor and therefore the binding of the ligand to the receptor does not alter the free (F) concentration of the ligand.
- The response elicited by receptor occupation is directly proportional to the number of receptors occupied by the ligand.

The equilibrium dissociation constant K_d gives a measure of the affinity of the ligand for the receptor.

$$K_d = ([R][L]) / [RL] \qquad\qquad (2.20)$$

K_d can also be defined by the two microconstants for rate on and off k_{+1} and k_{-1} so that $K_d = k_{-1} / k_{+1}$, where K_d is the concentration of the ligand (L) that occupies 50% of the available receptors.

Antagonist ligands occupy the receptor without eliciting a response, thus preventing agonist ligands from producing their effects. Since this interaction is usually competitive in nature, an agonist can overcome the antagonist effects as its concentration is increased. The competitive nature of this interaction allows the determination of a pA_2 value, the affinity of an antagonist for a receptor as shown below.

$$pA_2 = -\log K_B \qquad\qquad (2.21)$$

where K_B = the dissociation constant for a competitive antagonist, and is the ligand concentration that occupies 50% of the receptors.

We thus have a series of unbound drug affinity measures relating to the action of the drug. The values are those typically obtained by the pharmacologist and form the basis of the structure–activity relationships the medicinal chemist will work on. It is possible to extend this model to provide a pharmacokinetic phase as shown in Fig. 2.9.

Here we assume that:
1. The free drug is in equilibrium across the system.
2. Only the free drug can exert pharmacological activity (see above).
3. Drug is reversibly bound to tissues and blood.
4. Only the free drug can be cleared.

To examine the validity of this model, data from a number of seven transmembrane (7TM) receptor antagonists (antimuscarinics, antihistaminics, β-adrenoceptor blockers, etc.) were examined. The K_B values for these drugs were compared to

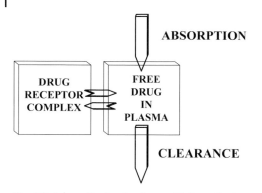

Fig. 2.9 Schematic showing the equilibrium of a drug receptor and unbound (free) drug and the processes that control drug concentration.

their free (unbound) plasma concentration. To simplify the analysis the plasma concentration data was taken from patients at steady state on therapeutic doses. Steady state means that the dosing rate (rate in) is balanced by the clearance rate (rate out). This concept is exactly as described earlier for intravenous infusion; however, the steady state is an average of the various peaks and troughs that occur in a normal dosage regimen. The relationship between the values was very close, by adjustment of the *in vitro* potency values to 75% receptor occupancy (*RO*) rather than 50% by Eq. 2.22 shown below (where the ligand concentration is represented by L):

$$RO = [L] / [K_B + L] \tag{2.22}$$

When this relationship is plotted, a 1:1 relationship is seen, as shown in Fig. 2.10. Thus the free concentration present in plasma is that actually seen at the receptor.

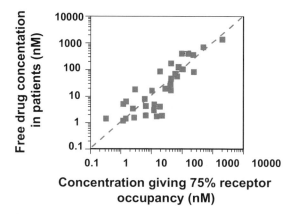

Fig. 2.10 Correlation of *in vitro* potency with plasma free drug concentration required for efficacy.

Moreover, the *in vitro* values (K_B) determined from receptor binding actually represent a concentration needed in the patient for efficacy.

We can thus see that the traditional indicators of potency that drive synthetic chemistry, such as pA_2 values, can have direct relevance to the plasma concentration (free) required to elicit the required response. If we extend this example further it is unlikely that in all cases there is a simple direct equilibrium for all compounds between the free drug in plasma and the aqueous media bathing the receptor. The free concentration of drug in the plasma is in direct equilibrium with the interstitial fluid bathing most cells of the body, since the capillary wall contains sufficient pores to allow the rapid passage of relatively small molecules, regardless of physicochemistry. Most receptor targets are accessed extracellularly. We can expect therefore that all drugs, regardless of their physicochemistry, will be in direct equilibrium at these targets, with the free drug in plasma. For instance the G-protein coupled receptors have a binding site which is accessible to hydrophilic molecules.

This is exemplified by the endogenous agonists of these receptors that are usually hydrophilic by nature. Adrenaline, dopamine and histamine are representative and have log $D_{7.4}$ values of -2.6, -2.4 and -2.9, respectively.

The antagonists included in Fig. 2.10 range in log $D_{7.4}$ value. For example, within the β-adrenoceptor antagonists the range is from -1.9 for atenolol to 1.1 for propranolol. This range indicates the ease of passage from the circulation to the receptor site for both hydrophilic and lipophilic drugs.

2.10
Unbound Drug Model and Barriers to Equilibrium

In some cases barriers such as the blood-brain barrier exist, in other cases the target is intracellular. Here the model has to be extended to place the receptor in a biophase (Fig. 2.11). The model also includes a *compartment* for a drug that is re-

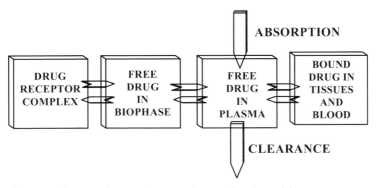

Fig. 2.11 Schematic pharmacodynamic/pharmacokinetic model incorporating a biophase and a drug binding compartment.

versibly bound to tissues and blood. The significance of this will be explored after further examination of the role of the biophase.

Aqueous channels are much fewer in number in the capillaries of the brain (blood-brain barrier) and rapid transfer into the brain fluids requires molecules to traverse the lipid cores of the membranes. Actual passage into cells, like crossing the blood-brain barrier, also requires molecules to transit the lipid core of the membrane due to the relative paucity of aqueous channels. Distribution to the target for a drug, whether a cell membrane receptor in the CNS or an intracellular enzyme or receptor, therefore critically determines the range of physicochemical properties available for the drug discoverer to exploit. The access of the CNS to drugs is illustrated by reference to a series of dopamine D_2 antagonists. Here receptor occupancy can be measured by the use of PET scanning and this *direct measure* of receptor occupancy can be compared with theoretical occupation calculated from the free drug plasma concentrations in the same experiment. Figure 2.12 shows this comparison for the lipophilic antagonists remoxipride, clozapine, haloperidol and thioridazine, and the hydrophilic compound sulpiride.

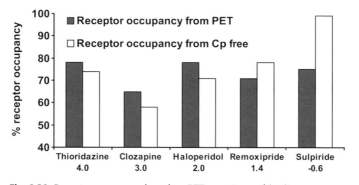

Fig. 2.12 Receptor occupancy based on PET scanning and *in vitro* potency combined with free plasma drug concentration. Log $D_{7.4}$ values shown below compound names.

As for the more comprehensive set of non-CNS site antagonists, referred to above, efficacy is observed around 75% receptor occupancy. Noticeably, the lipophilic antagonists thioridazine, clozapine, haloperidol and remoxipride, are in direct equilibrium with the free drug concentration in plasma. In contrast sulpiride requires a free plasma concentration over 50-fold greater than that required if there was a simple direct equilibrium between the plasma concentration and the extracellular fluid of the brain. This difference in equilibrium between sulpiride and the lipophilic compounds is due to the poor penetration of this hydrophilic molecule across the blood-brain barrier. As explained above, the reasons for this are the low number of aqueous channels or pores at the capillary wall of the blood vessels of the brain, thereby restricting entry of hydrophilic compounds to the extracellular fluid of the CNS. Similar observations can be made for intracellular targets, whether enzymes or receptors. Here the need to penetrate the lipid core is reflected in the physicochemistry of the endogenous agonists. For instance, steroid receptors are intracellular and steroids have log $D_{7.4}$ values such as 3.3, 1.7 and 2.3 for testosterone, cortisol and corticosterone, respectively. These values contrast with the values for the endogenous agonists of G-protein coupled receptors.

2.11
Slow Offset Compounds

One frequently encounters the case when the equilibrium dissociation constant (K_d, see Section 2.9) is defined by microconstants with *fast* rates on and off the receptor. However, any change in potency in a chemical series (affinity) must represent an increase in the on (k_{+1}) rate or a decrease in the off rate (k_{-1}). Occasionally, either by accident or design, the off rate is altered dramatically enough to redefine the receptor kinetics of the compound such that the rates influence the actual pharmacodynamics of the compound. These compounds are termed *slow offset* and their pharmacodynamic action exceeds that which would be predicted from the duration of the plasma concentrations. Often such compounds are detected during *in vitro* studies by increasing affinity or potency with time of incubation or persistence of activity following removal of the drug by *wash out*. A number of explanations for this phenomena have been advanced. Extra-receptor binding attempts to explain the slow offset of a compound by invoking a binding site removed from the actual active site domain. This site could be either protein or lipid. Salmeterol (a β2-adrenoceptor agonist) represents an agent designed in this manner [10]. The lipophilic side chain interacts with an exosite and markedly improves duration against compounds such as salbutamol (Fig. 2.13).

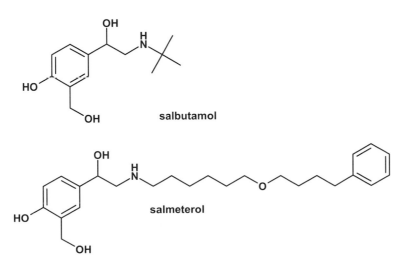

salbutamol

salmeterol

Fig. 2.13 Structures of salbutamol and salmeterol, rapid and slow offset β2-adrenoceptor agonists.

The exosite appears to be located at the interface of the cytoplasm and the transmembrane domain of the β2-adrenergic receptor [10]. The structures of salbutamol and salmeterol are clearly different, although it is obvious both are based on the adrenalin pharmacophore. More subtle changes in structure leading to slow-offset can only be rationalised by changes in intrareceptor binding. Possibilities for such increases can include simply increased interaction per se and resultant affinity, with an effect largely confined to changes in the off rate. Thus, telenzepine is more potent than pirenzepine as well as showing slow offset from the receptor [11]. This increase in affinity may simply reflect the increased lipophilicity of the telenzepine head group (Fig. 2.14).

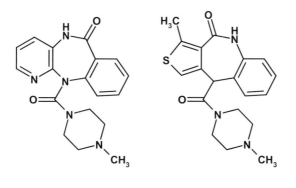

pirenzepine   **telenzepine**

Fig. 2.14 Structures of pirenzepine and its more potent, slow offset M1 antimuscarinic analogue telenzepine.

It is possible to achieve slow offset without a change in potency. Here conformational restriction may be the mechanism. If one assumes a number of binding functions in a molecule, and that for stable binding all have to interact, then probability suggests that in a flexible molecule association and disassociation will be

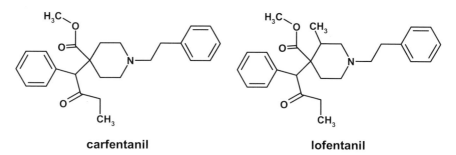

carfentanil   **lofentanil**

Fig. 2.15 Structures of opioid agonists carfentanil and its slow offset analogue lofentanil.

occurring rapidly (fast on, fast off). With a molecule whose confirmation is restricted to one favourable to the interactions, it is likely that the rate of association and dissociation will be markedly lower (slow on, slow off). Such restrictions may be very simple molecular changes, for instance a single methyl group converts the fast offset compound carfentanil [12] to the slow offset compound lofentanil (Fig. 2.15).

2.12
Factors Governing Unbound Drug Concentration

We thus have in many cases only two parameters defining drug activity at steady state, receptor affinity and free (unbound) plasma concentration. Occasionally actual persistence at the receptor needs to be taken into account. In some cases, particularly hydrophilic drugs, there is a permeation factor that needs to be defined. The concept of steady state allows simplification of the equations and concepts of pharmacokinetics. Steady state in the context here implies a drug dosed at specific times so that the concentrations between administered doses are effectively an exact image of previous doses and that the difference between the peak and trough levels are small. The factors governing the steady state free plasma concentration $C_{p(f)}$, for an oral drug, are the dosing rate (dose multiplied by frequency), the fraction of the dose absorbed (F_{da}) through the GIT and the free drug clearance (Cl_u) as shown below:

at steady state: rate in = rate out

$$(\text{Dose} \times \text{Frequency}) \times F = C_{p(f)} \times Cl_u \qquad (2.23)$$

True steady state is usually only achieved for a prolonged period with intravenous infusion. If we assume that we wish for a similar steady value after oral administration, then we need to balance our dosing frequency with the rate of decline of drug concentration, and the rule of thumb referred to earlier (dosing interval equal to drug half-life) can be applied. Unbound clearance and the free drug are particularly applicable to drugs delivered by the oral route. For a well-absorbed compound the free plasma concentrations directly relate to Cl_{iu} (intrinsic unbound clearance).

$$\text{AUC} = \text{Dose} / Cl_{iu} \qquad (2.24)$$

This simplifies greatly the concepts of first-pass hepatic metabolism and systemic clearance referred to previously. Most importantly Cl_{iu} is directly evolved from the enzyme kinetic parameters, V_{max} and K_m:

$$Cl_{iu} = V_{max} / K_m \qquad (2.25)$$

When the drug concentrations are below the K_m, Cl_{iu} is essentially independent of drug concentration. The processes of drug metabolism are similar to other enzymatic processes. For instance most oxidative processes (cytochrome P450) obey Michaelis–Menten kinetics:

$$v = [V_{max} \cdot s] / [K_m + s] \tag{2.26}$$

where v is the rate of the reaction, V_{max} the maximum rate, K_m the affinity constant (concentration at 50% V_{max}) and s the substrate concentration. Substrate concentration (s) is equal to or has a direct relationship to $C_{p(f)}$. In many cases $C_{p(f)}$ (or s) are below the K_m value of the enzyme system. However, in some cases (particularly the higher affinity P450s such as CYP2D6, see metabolic clearance), $C_{p(f)}$ (or s) can exceed the K_m and the rate of metabolism therefore approaches the maximum (V_{max}). As such, the kinetics move from first order to zero order and the elimination of the drug is capacity limited. The term saturation kinetics is applied. Under these conditions

$$Cl_{iu} = V_{max} / s \tag{2.27}$$

and clearance depends on drug concentration.

These values are obtained from *in vitro* enzyme experiments. From the previous relationship between *in vitro* pharmacology measurements, free drug concentrations, and the ones outlined here, it is reasonable to assume that clinical dose size can be calculated from simple *in vitro* measurements.

It is easiest to understand how clearance relates to the rate of decline of drug concentration (half-life) if we consider the model depicted in Fig. 2.9. When a dose (D) is administered intravenously then the initial free concentration in plasma achieved $C_{p(fo)}$ is dependant on volume of extracellular or total body water minus plasma water and the amount of drug bound to tissues and proteins.

Free volume is calculated by equations analogous to those for total drug (see Eq. 2.1).

$$C_{p(fo)} = D / V_{d(f)} \tag{2.28}$$

in which $V_{d(f)}$ is an apparent volume not only including the actual fluid the drug is dissolved in but also including the drug bound to tissues and protein as if it was an aqueous compartment in direct equilibrium with the free drug. Thus, the greater the amount of drug bound the greater the apparent free volume. The clearance and volume of distribution of an unbound drug are related by the equation

$$Cl_u = V_{d(f)} \times k_{el} \tag{2.29}$$

where k_{el} is the elimination rate constant. Note that this equation and others are essentially the same as those for total drug other than free (unbound) drug values substituted for total drug values. Free volume and free clearance are always equal to or greater than the values calculated from the total drug. Moreover, increases in plasma protein binding increase free volume but decrease total volume.

These concepts lead to two important observations. Protein binding or tissue binding is not important in daily dose size. The daily dose size is determined by the required free (unbound) concentration of drug required for efficacy. Protein binding or tissue binding is important in actual dosage regimen (frequency). The greater the binding the lower and more sustained the free drug concentrations are. Thus a drug with fourfold higher binding, and hence larger free volume than another, with the same unbound (free) clearance, will have a fourfold longer half-life. This could result in a dosage regimen of 20 mg once a day compared to 5 mg four times a day, both giving rise to broadly similar profiles and fluctuations around the average steady state concentration.

References

1 Haller, M., Akbulut, C., Brechtelsbauer, H., Fett, W., Briegel, J., Finsterer, U., Peter, K. **1993**, *Life Sci.* 53, 1597–1604.

2 Burns, E., Triger, D.R., Tucker, G.T., Bax, N.D.S. **1991**, *Clin. Sci.* 80, 155–160.

3 Wong, W.W., Sheng, H.P., Morkeberg, J.C., Kosanovich, J.L., Clarke, L.L., Klein, P.D. **1989**,. *Am. J. Clin. Nutr.* 50, 1290–1294.

4 Brans, Y.W., Kazzi, N.J., Andrew, D.S., Schwartz, C.A., Carey, K.D. **1990**, *Biol. Neonate* 58, 137–144.

5 Gibaldi, M., McNamara, P.J. **1978**, *Eur. J. Clin. Pharmacol,* 13, 373–378.

6 Stopher, D.A., Beresford, A.P., Macrae, P.V., Humphrey, M.J. **1988**, *J. Cardiovasc. Pharmacol.* 12, S55–S59.

7 Edgar, B., Regardh, C.G., Johnsson, G., Johansson, L., Lundborg, P., Loftberg, I., Ronn, O. **1985**, *Clin. Pharmacol. Ther.* 38, 205–211.

8 Smith, D.A., Rasmussen, H.S., Stopher, D.A., Walker, D.K. **1992**, *Xenobiotica* 22, 709–719.

9 Thummel, K.E., Kunze, K.L., Shen, D.D. **1997**, *Adv. Drug Delivery Rev.* 27, 99–127.

10 Green, S.A., Spasoff, A.P., Coleman, R.A., Johnson, M., Liggett, S.B. **1996**, *J. Biol. Chem.* 271, 24029–24035.

11 Schudt, C., Auriga, C., Kinder, B., Birdsall, N.J.M. **1988**, *Eur. J. Pharmacol* 145, 87–90.

12 Leysen, J.E., Gommeren, W. **1986**, *Drug Dev. Res.* 8, 119–131.

3
Absorption

3.1
The Absorption Process

The oral absorption of a drug is dependant on the compound dissolving in the aqueous contents of the gastrointestinal tract (dissolution) and then traversing the actual barrier of the gastrointestinal tract to reach the blood (Fig. 3.1). For a number of reasons membrane transfer may be limited (see Fig. 3.2) and therefore absorption incomplete. In this chapter these processes will be discussed.

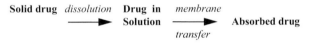

Fig. 3.1 Simplified view of the absorption process.

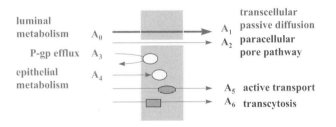

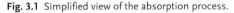

$$A\% = -a_0A_0 + a_1A_1 + a_2A_2 - a_3A_3 - a_4A_4 + a_5A_5 + a_6A_6$$

Fig. 3.2 Mechanisms of membrane permeation [1]. The total percentage of the dose absorbed may the result of a combination of several of these processes.

Pharmacokinetics and Metabolism in Drug Design.
Dennis A. Smith, Han van de Waterbeemd, Don K. Walker (Eds.)
Copyright © 2006 WILEY-VCH Verlag GmbH & Co. KGaA, Weinheim
ISBN: 3-527-31368-0

3.2
Dissolution

Dissolution depends on the surface area of the dissolving solid and the solubility of the drug at the surface of the dissolving solid. Considering these factors separately, surface area is manipulated by the processing and formulation of the compound. Milling and micronisation form the drug into smaller particles with consequently increase surface area. In actual clinical use the compaction of the particles into tablets is offset by formulation with disintegrants. Certain formulations use a co-solvent such as polyethylene glycol (PEG), which is an organic solvent with water miscible properties.

Solubility is manipulated mainly by the structure of the drug. Broadly, solubility is inversely proportional to the number and type of lipophilic functions within the molecule and the tightness of the crystal packing of the molecule. Yalkowski [2] has produced a general solubility (log S) equation, for organic non-electrolytes. The equation incorporates the entropy of melting (ΔS_m) and melting point (*mp* in °C) as a measure of crystal packing, and log P as a measure of lipophilicity.

$$\log S = [S_m \, (mp - 25) \, / \, 1364] - \log P + 0.80 \tag{3.1}$$

This equation can be further simplified to

$$\log S = - \log P - 0.01 \, mp + 1.2 \tag{3.2}$$

It can be seen from the above that increases in either crystal packing or lipophilicity will decrease solubility.

The rate of dissolution is effected by solubility, as is the actual concentration of the drug in the bulk of the solution (aqueous contents of gastrointestinal tract). Concentration of the drug in solution is the driving force of the membrane transfer of the drug into the body, and low aqueous solubility often continues to present itself as a problem even after formulation improvements.

A number of drugs have very low aqueous solubility, mainly due to very high lipophilicity, but also due to lack of ionisable centre, and also the tight crystal packing referred to above. These drugs are erratically and incompletely absorbed due to this inability to dissolve in the gastrointestinal tract following oral administration. Examples of low solubility, dissolution-limited drugs include danazol, griseofulvin, halofantrine, ketoconazole, nitrofurantoin, phenytoin and triamterene [3, 4]. Poor dissolution is responsible for both intra- and interpatient variability in drug absorption, and so represents a major problem in drug design.

If a drug has an ionisable centre then solubility can be improved by salt formation. In the absence of a salt basic drugs will also have increased solubility in the acidic environment of the stomach.

The incorporation of an ionisable centre, such as an amine or similar function, into a template can bring a number of benefits including water solubility. A key step in the discovery of indinavir was the incorporation of a basic amine (and a

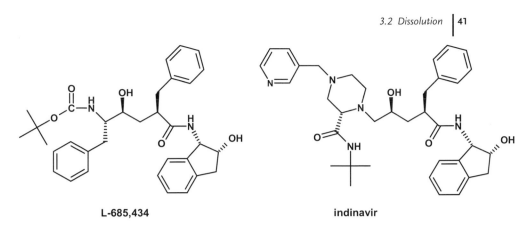

L-685,434   **indinavir**

Fig. 3.3 Structures of lead compound L-685,434 and indinavir which
incorporates basic functions aiding water solubility.

pyridine) into the backbone of hydroxyethylene transition state mimic compounds
(Fig. 3.3) to enhance solubility (and potency) [5].

A particular problem in drug discovery is that solubility is not constant. When a
newly synthesised compound is first isolated it is often as the amorphous form.
In this form solubility is invariably at its highest. Subsequent isolation will be in a
crystalline form and a decrease in solubility is seen. As purification (crystallisation) conditions are improved further, polymorphs are isolated, each representing
the thermodynamically most stable form. Polymorphs are different crystalline
forms, which although chemically identical, result from a different ordered
arrangement of molecules within the crystalline lattice. This process of crystals
with increasing thermodynamic stability and resultant lower solubility if referred
to as Ostwald's *rule of stages*. This rule or law states that when leaving a given state
and in transforming to another state, the state which is sought out is not the thermodynamically stable one, but the state nearest in stability to the original state.
This rule therefore implies that the first solid formed in crystallisation will be the
least stable polymorph and the one with the largest Gibbs free energy. The rule is
certainly not a law, for instance, solvents, rendering the sequence of crystallisation
depends on which solvent is first tried. Similarly, the formation of hydrates can be
dependent on the water concentration of the crystallising solvent. Although not a
hard and fast principle, early solubility data on discovery or event early development compounds should be viewed with caution, since there is a strong chance
that it will decrease. Another issue is that solubility is strongly dependent on the
medium and experimental conditions including pH, ionic strength, and buffer
(see also Chapter 1). Therefore solubility in pure water is often different from solubility in, e.g. artificial GI fluid.

The discovery of a less soluble polymorph can even occur post-launch. Ritonavir
was discovered in 1992, had a new drug application filed in 1995 and subsequently introduced to the market as a semisolid formulation. In 1998 a polymorph, form II, *appeared* causing failure of many final product lots due to poorer
dissolution; the form being much less soluble in the formulation solvents.

3.3
Membrane Transfer

The barrier of the gastrointestinal tract is similar to any other that involves the crossing of biological membranes. Biomembranes are composed of a lipid bilayer [6]. The bilayer results from the orientation of the lipids (phospholipids, glycolipids and cholesterol) in the aqueous medium. Phospholipids are amphipathic with polar head groups and lipid *tails*, and align so that the polar head groups orientate to the aqueous medium and the lipid tails form an inner hydrophobic core. Because of the high flexibility of the membrane lipids they are able to perform transversal/lateral movements within the membrane. In the membrane different proteins are embedded such as selective ion channels (Na^+, K^+, Ca^{2+}, Cl^-). Tight junctions are formed by the interaction of membrane proteins at the contact surfaces between single cells. Tight junctions are in reality small aqueous filled pores. The dimensions of these pores have been estimated to be in the range of 3–10 Å. The number and dimensions of the tight junctions depends on the membrane type. For the small intestine it amounts about 0.01% of the whole surface. Thus the surface area of the actual biological membrane is much greater than the aqueous pores (tight junctions).

Compounds can cross biological membranes by two passive processes, transcellular and paracellular. For transcellular diffusion two potential mechanisms exist. The compound can distribute into the lipid core of the membrane and diffuse within the membrane to the basolateral side. Alternatively, the solute may diffuse across the apical cell membrane and enter the cytoplasm before exiting across the basolateral membrane. Because both processes involve diffusion through the lipid core of the membrane, the physicochemistry of the compound is important. Paracellular absorption involves the passage of the compound through the aqueous filled pores. Clearly, in principle, many compounds can be absorbed by this route but the process is invariably slower than transcellular (surface area of pores *versus* surface area of the membrane) and is very dependant on molecular size due to the finite dimensions of the aqueous pores.

The actual amount of a drug absorbed (F_a) is dependent on two rates: the rate of absorption (k_a) and the rate of disappearance of the drug from the absorption site. The disappearance can be due to absorption (k_a) or movement of the drug (k_m) through the gastrointestinal tract and away from the absorption site. The proportion absorbed can be written as:

$$F_a = k_a / (k_a + k_m) \tag{3.3}$$

Compounds crossing the gastrointestinal tract via the transcellular route can usually be absorbed throughout the length of the tract. In contrast, the paracellular route is only readily available in the small intestine and the term absorption window is often applied. The calculated human pore sizes (radii) are jejunum 6–8 Å, ileum 2.9–3.8 Å and colon less than 2.3 Å. In practice the small intestine transit time is around six hours, whilst transit of the whole tract is approximately twenty-four hours. For lipophilic compounds, with adequate dissolution, which have high rates of transcellular passage across membranes, k_a is a high value. Moreover, since the drug is absorbed throughout the GI tract k_m is of a low value and therefore the proportion of a dose absorbed is high (complete). For hydrophilic compounds, which are dependent on the slow paracellular pathway, k_a is a low value. Moreover, the absorption window means that the drug rapidly moves away from the absorption site and k_m is high. Consequently paracellularly absorbed compounds show incomplete absorption with the proportion absorbed low. Table 3.1 gives examples of compounds absorbed by the paracellular route.

Tab. 3.1 Examples of drugs absorbed by the paracellular route.

Compound	Log $D_{7.4}$	Molecular weight	% Absorbed
Nadolol	−2.1	309	13
Sotalol	−1.7	272	100
Atenolol	−1.5	266	51
Practolol	−1.3	266	100
Xamoterol	−1.0	339	9
Amosulalol	−0.8	380	100
Sumatriptan	−0.8	295	60
Pirenzipine	−0.6	351	25
Famotidine	−0.6	338	37
Ranitidine	−0.3	314	50

What is noticeable is that the compounds are of low molecular weight; however, their is no simple relationship between molecular weight and percent absorbed, probably indicating that shape and possibly flexibility are also of importance. Related compounds such as propranolol (log $D_{7.4} = 0.9$) to those in Table 3.1 show high flux rates via the transcellular route and consequently complete absorption. Note, however, that lipophilicity correlates with increased metabolic lability and such compounds may have their apparent systemic availabilities decreased by metabolism as they pass through the gut and the liver.

For simple molecules, like β-adrenoceptor antagonists octanol/water log $D_{7.4}$ values are remarkably predictive of absorption potential. Compounds with log $D_{7.4}$ values below zero are absorbed predominantly by the paracellular route and compounds with log $D_{7.4}$ values above zero are absorbed by the transcellular route.

Another example of the relationship between log D values and intestinal absorption is taken from [1] (see Fig. 3.4). Compounds with log D greater than zero demonstrate a nearly complete absorption. Two exceptions are compounds with a MW above 500. If size as such, or the accompanying increase in the number of H-bonds is responsible for poorer absorption is not fully understood.

However, as the number of H-bonding functions in a molecule rises, octanol/water distribution, in isolation, becomes a progressively less valuable predictor.

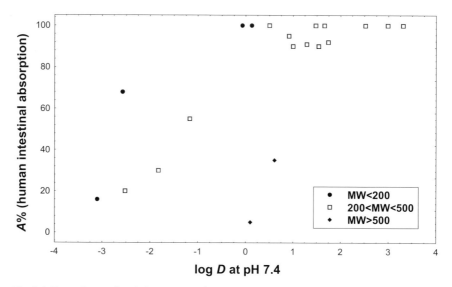

Fig. 3.4 Dependence of oral absorption on log D [1].

For such compounds desolvation and breaking of H-bonds becomes the rate-limiting step in transfer across the membrane [7].

Methods to calculate H-bonding potential range from simple H-bond counts (number of donors and acceptors), through systems that assign a value of one for donors and 0.5 for acceptors to sophisticated scoring systems such as the Raevsky H-bond score [8]. The correlation of Raevsky H-bond scores with Δlog D, shown previously as Fig. 1.4, is shown below as Fig. 3.5.

None of these methods gives a perfect prediction, particularly because H-bonding potential needs to be layered over intrinsic lipophilicity. For this reason Lipinski's *rule of five* becomes valuable as defining the outer limits in which chemists can work [9]. Lipinski defined the boundaries of good absorption potential by demonstrating that poor permeability is produced by:

1. more than five H-bond donors (sum of OH and NH);
2. more than ten H-bond acceptors (sum of N and O);
3. molecular weight over 500;
4. poor dissolution by log P over five.

The medicinal chemist can use these rules and understand the boundaries and work to lowering these values. Figure 3.6 shows a synthetic strategy aimed at removing H-bond donors from a series of endothelin antagonists and a resultant increase in apparent bioavailability as determined by intraduodenal AUC [10]. Noticeable CLOGP values vary only marginally with the changes in structure, val-

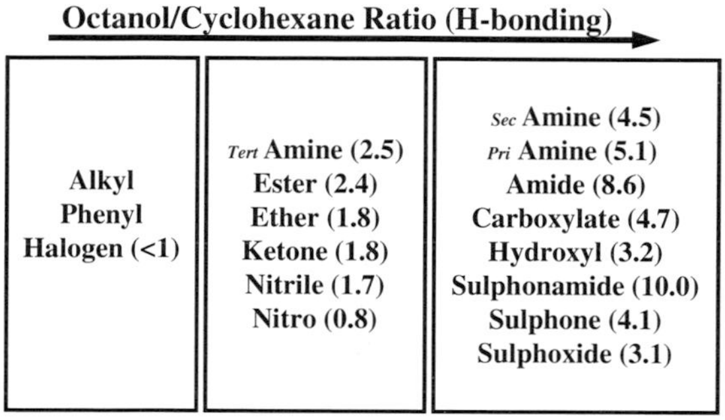

Octanol/Cyclohexane Ratio (H-bonding)

Alkyl Phenyl Halogen (<1)	*Tert* Amine (2.5) Ester (2.4) Ether (1.8) Ketone (1.8) Nitrile (1.7) Nitro (0.8)	*Sec* Amine (4.5) *Pri* Amine (5.1) Amide (8.6) Carboxylate (4.7) Hydroxyl (3.2) Sulphonamide (10.0) Sulphone (4.1) Sulphoxide (3.1)

Fig. 3.5 Raevsky H-bond scores from HYBOT95 (shown in brackets) and correlation with Δlog *D* (compare with Fig. 1.4).

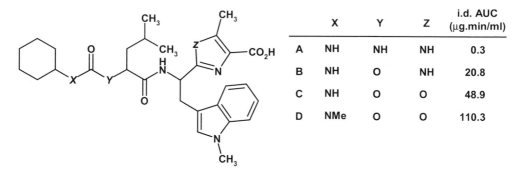

	X	Y	Z	i.d. AUC (μg.min/ml)
A	NH	NH	NH	0.3
B	NH	O	NH	20.8
C	NH	O	O	48.9
D	NMe	O	O	110.3

Fig. 3.6 Removal of H-bond donors as a synthetic strategy for a series of azole-containing endothelin antagonists aimed at improving bioavailability by lowering H-bonding potential [10].

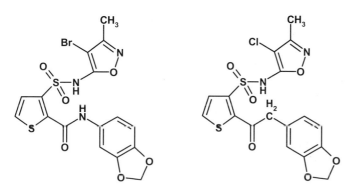

Fig. 3.7 Replacement of amide with acetyl in a series of amidothiophene-sulfonamide endothelin-A antagonists to improve oral bioavailability [11].

ues being 4.8, 5.0, 4.8 and 5.5 for compounds A, B, C and D, respectively. In contrast the number of H-bond donors is reduced by three and the Raevsky score from 28.9 (A) to 21.4 (D).

A similar example, also from endothelin antagonists, is the replacement of the amide group (Fig. 3.7) in a series of amidothiophenesulfonamides with acetyl [11]. This move retained *in vitro* potency, but markedly improved oral bioavailability.

3.4
Barriers to Membrane Transfer

The cells of the gastrointestinal tract contain a number of enzymes of drug metabolism and also various transport proteins. Of particular importance in the attenuation of absorption/bioavailability are the glucuronyl and sulphotransferases, which metabolise phenol containing drugs sufficiently rapidly to attenuate the passage of the intact drug across the gastrointestinal tract. Cytochrome P450 enzymes are also present, in particular CYP3A4 (see Chapter 7), and again certain substrates for the drug may be metabolised during passage across the tract. This effect may be greatly enhanced by the action of the efflux pumps, in particular P-glycoprotein. P-glycoprotein's range of substrates is large but includes a number of relatively large molecular weight drugs which are also CYP3A4 substrates. Cyclosporine A is one example. This drug shows significant attenuation of absorption across the gastrointestinal tract due to metabolism. The metabolism by the gut is greater than many other examples of CYP3A4 substrates. It can be postulated that in effect absorption of the drug is followed by secretion back into the lumen of the gut by P-glycoprotein. This cyclical process effectively exposes cyclosporin A to *multi-pass* metabolism by CYP3A4, resulting in a lower appearance of intact cyclosporin A in the circulation.

Detailed structure–activity relationships of P-glycoprotein are not yet available. Some understanding is provided by Seelig [12] who has compared structural features in P-glycoprotein substrates. This analysis has indicated that recognition elements are present in structures and are formed by two (type I) or three electron donor groups (type II) with a fixed spatial separation. The type I element consists of two electron donor groups separated by 2.5 Å, whilst the type II elements have a spatial separation of the outer groups by 4.6 Å. All molecules that are P-glycoprotein substrates contain at least one of these groups and the affinity of the substrate for P-glycoprotein depends on the strength and number of electron donor or hydrogen bond acceptor groups. For the purpose of this analysis, all groups with an unshared electron pair on an electronegative atom (O, N, S or F and Cl), or groups with a π-electron orbital of an unsaturated system, were considered as electron donors. However, this analysis did not account for the directionality of the H-bonds.

The dramatic effect of a single unit is shown in Fig. 3.8 for a series of β-adrenoceptor antagonists.

	E (g i)	E(h)

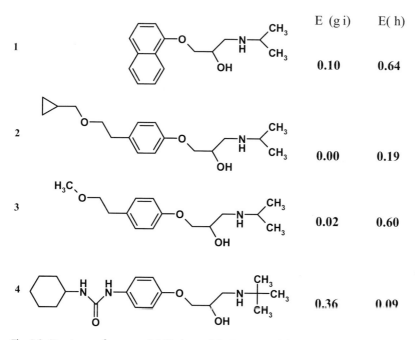

1   0.10   0.64

2   0.00   0.19

3   0.02   0.60

4   0.36   0.09

Fig. 3.8 Structures of propranolol (1), betaxolol (2), metoprolol (3) and talinolol (4) and their respective extraction by the gastrointestinal tract E(GI) and liver E(h).

All these compounds are moderately lipophilic and should show excellent ability to cross biological membranes (transcellular absorption). Propranolol, betaxolol and metoprolol all have minimal gut first-pass metabolism, as shown by the low value for E(GI). Metabolism and first-pass effects for these compounds are largely confirmed to the liver as shown by the values for E(GI). In contrast, talinolol shows a large extraction by the gastrointestinal tract with a low liver extraction [13]. These effects are illustrated graphically in Fig. 3.9, which shows the bioavail-

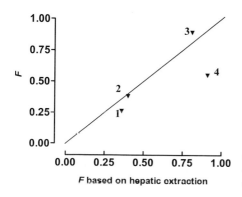

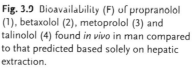

Fig. 3.9 Bioavailability (F) of propranolol (1), betaxolol (2), metoprolol (3) and talinolol (4) found *in vivo* in man compared to that predicted based solely on hepatic extraction.

ability predicted from hepatic extraction contrasted with the obtained *in vivo* in man.

Noticeably propranolol, betaxolol and metoprolol are close or on the line for hepatic first-pass effects, whereas talinolol falls markedly below it. Talinolol has been shown to be a substrate for P-glycoprotein [14]. The effect of the urea function is of key importance within this change, the urea acting as a strong type I unit in terms of Seelig's classification. Other changes in the molecule, such as the tertiary butyl, rather than isopropyl N-substituent are not so important since the

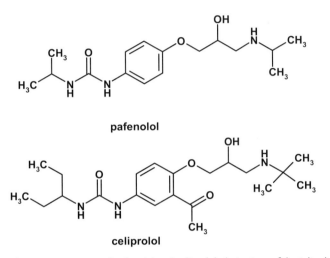

pafenolol

celiprolol

Fig. 3.10 Structures of pafenolol and celiprolol, derivatives of the talinolol (see Fig. 3.6) structure which show similar bioavailability characteristics.

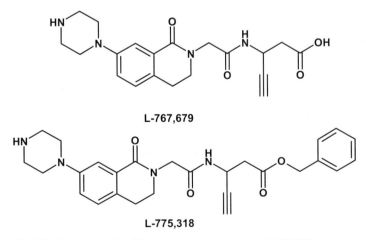

L-767,679

L-775,318

Fig. 3.11 Structures of the fibrinogen receptor antagonist L-767,679 and its benzyl ester (L-775,318) analogue.

related compounds pafenolol and celiprolol (Fig. 3.10) also show similar bioavail-ability features.

These considerations are important in prodrug design and add to the complex-ity referred to earlier. Many active principles in prodrug programmes are non-lipo-philic compounds, possessing a number of H-bond donor and acceptor functions (amide or peptide linkages). Addition of a pro-moiety will raise the lipophilicity and molecular weight. In doing so, the final molecule may have the characteristics to traverse the lipid core of a membrane, but this advantage is lost by it becoming a substrate for efflux. An example (Fig. 3.11) of this is the fibrinogen receptor antagonist L-767,679, a low lipophilicity compound (log $P < -3$) with resultant low membrane flux. The benzyl ester (L-775,318) analogue (log P 0.7) also showed limited absorption, and studies in Caco-2 cells (see Section 3.5) showed the com-pound to be effluxed by P-glycoprotein [15].

3.5
Models for Absorption Estimation

A number of models have been suggested to estimate the absorption potential of new compounds in humans (see Table 3.2) [16, 17, 17a]. These vary from low-throughput (*in situ* rat model) to high-throughput (*in silico*) models. Most compa-nies will use a combination of these approaches.

The human colon adenocarcinoma cell lines Caco-2 and HT-29 are widely used as a screening model for absorption [18, 19]. An alternative is offered by the MDCK cell line was is a faster growing cell [20]. These cell lines have expression of typical impediments for absorption such the above-mentioned P-glycoprotein and CYP3A4 isoenzyme. They are thus believed to by a good mimic of the physi-cochemical and biological barrier of the GI tract.

More recently interest is growing to develop cheaper high-throughput evalua-tions of oral absorption since the cell-based systems are quite cost intensive. This resulted in systems such as the parallel artificial membrane permeability assay (PAMPA) developed by Kansy and colleagues [20a], as well as other alternatives based on the measurement of surface activity and surface plasmon resonance (SPR) [20b]. Increasingly, transporter-transfected cell lines are also being consid-ered to study the impact of transporter proteins on oral absorption, blood-brain penetration, and pharmacokinetics.

Tab. 3.2 *In vitro* screening for oral absorption/permeability.

Physicochemical profiling

Solubility
Ionisation (pK_a)
Lipophilicity
Octanol/water distribution/partitioning
Cyclohexane/water distribution/partitioning
Heptane/ethylene glycol distribution/partitioning
Immobilised artificial membranes (IAM)
Immobilised liposome chromatography (ILC)
Micellar electrokinetic chromatography (MEKC)
Biopartitioning micellar chromatography (BMC)
Hydrogen bonding
$\Delta\log P = \log P_{oct} - \log P_{alkane}$

Non-cell-based in vitro models

Phospholipid vesicles
Liposome partitioning
Impregnated artificial membranes
Parallel artificial membrane permeability assay (PAMPA)
Hexadecane-coated polycarbonate filters (HDM)
Transil particles
Surface plasmon resonance (SPR) biosensor
Surface activity

Cell-based in vitro models

Caco-2
MDCK
TC7
HT29
2/4/A1

Transporters and transfected cell lines

MDR1 (P-gp)
Calcein AM
Cycling
ATPase
MDCK-MDR1
MDCK-MRP2-OATP2
LLC-PK1–CYP3A

Ex vivo

Ussing chamber
Everted rings

In situ

Intestinal perfusion

3.6
Estimation of Absorption Potential

A simple dimensionless number, absorption potential (*AP*), has been proposed to make first approximation predictions of oral absorption (Eq. 3.4) [3].

$$AP = \log P + \log F_{non} + \log (S_o \cdot V_L/X_o) \qquad (3.4)$$

In this equation, $\log P$ is the partition coefficient for the neutral species, $\log F_{non}$ the fraction of non-ionised compound, S_o the intrinsic solubility, V_L the lumenal volume and X_o the given dose. By extending this approach also the effect of particle size on oral absorption has been modelled [21].

Considerable effort has been made to define what is acceptable solubility. The two key parameters that define this are permeability and dose size (potency), and these can be used to act as guidance to calculate an approximation of the maximum absorbable dose (*MAD*). An approach to estimate the maximum absorbable dose (*MAD*) in humans is based on Eq. 3.5 [22, 23].

$$MAD \text{ (mg)} = S_{6.5} \times k_a \times IFV \times RT \qquad (3.5)$$

Where S is the solubility in phosphate buffer at the pH 6.5 (in mg mL^{-1}), k_a the absorption rate constant in rats (in min^{-1}), *IFV* is the intestinal fluid volume (250 mL), and *RT* is the average residence time in the small intestine (270 min).

As a guide a compound with average permeability and a projected clinical dose of 100 mg needs an aqueous solubility of 50–100 µg mL^{-1}. A rule of thumb is that milligrams of clinical dose translate into µg mL^{-1} solubility. Note that pre-clinical safety and toxicity testing of such a compound may still be problematic due to the elevated dose levels probably required. The problem is compounded further by the *decreasing solubility* of crystalline and polymorphic forms, which may be encountered as the program continues.

3.7
Computational Approaches

As mentioned above, hydrogen bonding and molecular size, in combination with lipophilicity have an important influence on oral absorption. A number of methods are available to compute these properties [17a, 24–26]. An example of the correlation between H-bonding, expressed as polar surface area (*PSA*), and human oral absorption is found in Fig. 3.12 [27, 28]. Such a sigmoidal relationship is found for compounds which are absorbed by passive diffusion only and not hindered by efflux or metabolism, nor being involved in active uptake. Otherwise, deviations will be found [28].

Combination of several descriptors believed to be important for oral absorption have been used in various multivariate analysis studies [17a, 24]. The general

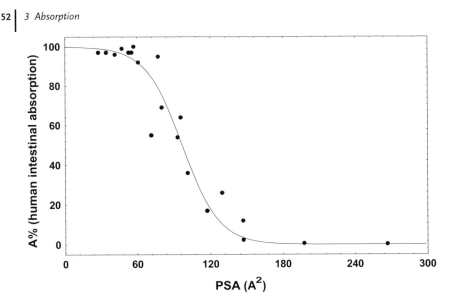

Fig. 3.12 Correlation between polar surface area (*PSA*) and intestinal absorption [27, 28].

trend is that a combination of a size/shape and a hydrogen-bond descriptor, sometimes in combination with log *D*, has good predictive value. At present time such models do not account for the biological function of the membrane, such as P-gp-mediated efflux and CYP3A4-mediated gut wall metabolism. Predictions form a cheap approach to early stage discovery screening for compounds with poor absorption potential.

References

1 Van de Waterbeemd, H. **1999**, Intestinal absorption: prediction from theory, in *Methods for Assessing Oral Drug Absorption*, Dressman, J. (ed.), Dekker, New York.

2 Yalkowski, S.H., Valvani, S.C. **1980**, *J. Pharm. Sci.* 69, 912–922.

3 Dressman, J.B., Amidon, G.L., Fleisher, D. **1985**, *J. Pharm. Sci.* 74, 588–589.

4 Amidon, G.L., Lennernas, H., Shah, V.P., Crison, J.R. **1995**, *Pharm. Res.* 12, 413–420.

5 Vacca, J.P., Dorsey, B.D., Schleif, W.A., Levin, R.B., McDaniel, S.L., Darke, P.L., Zugay, J., Quintero, J.C., Blahy, O.M., Roth, E., Sardana, V.V., Schlabach, A.J., Graham, P.I., Condra, J.H., Gotlib, L., Holloway, M.K., Lin, J., Chen, I.W., Vas-

tag, K., Ostovic, D., Anderson, P.S., Emini, E.A., Huff, J.R. **1994**, *Proc. Nat. Acad. Sci.* 91, 4096–4100.

6 Macheras, P., Reppas, C., Dressman, J.B. (eds.) **1995**, *Biopharmaceutics of Orally Administered Drugs*, Ellis Horwood, London.

7 Conradi, R.A., Burton, P.S., Borchardt, R.T. **1996**, Physicochemical and biological factors that influence a drug's cellular permeability by passive diffusion, in *Lipophilicity in Drug Action and Toxicology*, Pliska, V., Testa, B., Van de Waterbeemd, H. (eds.), VCH, Weinheim, (pp.) 233–252.

8 Raevsky, O.A., Grifor'er, V.Y., Kireev, D.B., Zefirov, N.S. **1992**, *Quant. Struct. Act. Relat.* 14, 433–436.

9 Lipinski, C.A., Lombardo, F., Dominy, B.W., Feeney, P.J. **1997**, *Adv. Drug Del. Revs.* 23, 3–25.

10 Von Geldern, T.W., Hoffman, D.J., Kester, J.A., Nellans, H.N., Dayton, B.D., Calzadilla, S.V., Marsch, K.C., Hernandez, L., Chiou W. **1996**, *J. Med. Chem.* 39, 982–991.

11 Wu, C., Chan, M.F., Stavros, F., Raju, B., Okun, I., Mong, S., Keller, K.M., Brock, T., Kogan, T.P., Dixon, R.A.F. **1997**, *J. Med. Chem.* 40, 1690–1697.

12 Seelig, A. **1998**, *Eur. Biochem.* 251, 252–261.

13 Travsch, B., Oertel, R., Richter, K., Gramatt, T. **1995**, *Biopharm. Drug Dispos.* 16, 403–414.

14 Spahn-Langguth, H., Baktir, G., Radschuweit, A., Okyar, A., Terhaag, B., Ader, P., Hanafy, A., Langguth, P. **1998**, *Int. J. Clin. Pharmacol. Ther.* 36, 16–24.

15 Prueksaitanont, T., Deluna, P., Gorham, L.M., Bennett, M.A., Cohn, D., Pang, J., Xu, X., Leung, K., Lin, J.H. **1998**, *Drug Met. Dispos.* 26, 520–527.

16 Borchardt, R.T., Smith, P.L., Wilson, G. (eds.) **1996**, *Models for Assessing Drug Absorption and Metabolism*, Plenum Press, New York.

17 Barthe, L., Woodley, J., Houin, G. **1999**, *Fundam. Clin. Pharmacol.* 13, 154–168.

17a Van de Waterbeemd, H., Models to predict oral absorption, in *Comprehensive Medicinal Chemistry*, Testa, B., Van de Waterbeemd, H. (eds.), 2nd ed, vol. 5, *ADMET Approaches*, Elsevier, Amsterdam, in press.

18 Hidalgo, I.J. **1996**, Cultured intestinal epithelial cell models, in *Models for Assessing Drug Absorption and Metabolism*, Borchardt, R.T., Smith, P.L., Wilson, G. (eds.), Plenum Press, New York, (pp.) 35–50.

19 Artursson, P., Palm, K., Luthman, K. **1996**, *Adv. Drug Deliv. Rev.* 22, 67–84.

20 Irvine, J.D., Takahashi, L., Lockhart, K., Cheong, J., Tolan, J.W., Selick, H.E., Grove, J.R. **1999**, *J. Pharm. Sci.* 88, 28–33.

20a Kansy, M., Avdeef, A., Fischer, H. **2004**, *Drug Disc. Today: Technol.* 1, 349–355.

20b Hämäläinen, M.D., Frostell-Karlsson, A. **2004**, *Drug Disc. Today: Technol.* 1, 397–404.

21 Oh, D.-M., Curl, R.L., Amidon, G.L. **1993**, *Pharm. Res.* 10, 264–270.

22 Johnson, K.C., Swindell, A.C. **1996**, *Pharm. Res.* 13, 1794–1797.

23 Lombardo, F., Winter, S.M., Tremain, L., Lowe, J.A. **1998**, The anxieties of drug discovery and development: CCK-B receptor antagonists, in *Integration of Pharmaceutical Discovery and Development: Case Studies*, Borchardt, R.T. et al. (eds.), Plenum Press, New York, (pp.) 465–479.

24 Van de Waterbeemd, H. **2000**, Quantitative structure-absorption relationships, in *Pharmacokinetic Optimization in Drug Research: Biological, Physicochemical and Computational Strategies*, Testa, B., Van de Waterbeemd, H., Folkers, G., Guy, R. (eds.), Verlag HCA, Basel, (pp.) 499–512.

25 Van de Waterbeemd, H., Jones, B.C. **2003**, *Progr. Med. Chem.* 41, 1–59.

26 Clark, D.E., Grootenhuis, P.D.J. **2003**, *Curr. Top. Med. Chem.* 2, 1193–1203.

27 Palm, K., Luthman, K., Ungell, A.-L., Strandlund, G., Beigi, F., Lundahl, P., Artursson, P. **1998**, *J. Med. Chem.* 41, 5382–5392.

28 Clark, D.E. **1999**, *J. Pharm. Sci.* 88, 807–814.

4
Distribution

4.1
Membrane Transfer Access to the Target

Distribution of drugs across the membranes of the body can be regarded as passive diffusion. Similar considerations to those already outlined for oral absorption apply, although for significant penetration to intracellular targets the aqueous pore pathway does not readily apply. Similarly, as previously outlined, the tight junctions of the capillaries supplying the CNS render the paracellular pathway very inefficient. These aspects of distribution were also described in the section concerning the unbound drug model and barriers to equilibrium. Figure 4.1 depicts a scheme for the distribution of drugs. Penetration from the circulation into the interstitial fluid is rapid for all drugs since the aqueous pores present in capillary membranes have a mean diameter of between 50–100 Å. Thus there is ready access to targets located at the surface of cells such as G-protein coupled receptors. The exception to this are the cerebral capillary network, since here there is a virtual absence of pores due to the continuous tight intercellular junction. For intracellular targets, if only the free drug is considered, then at steady state the concentrations present inside the cell and in the circulation should be similar for a drug that readily crosses the cell membrane.

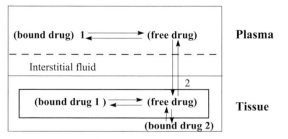

Fig. 4.1 Schematic illustrating drug distribution. Drug is present in the circulation as either free or bound; only the free drug is available to distribute; bound drug 1 in tissues is the drug bound to intracellular proteins and constituents; bound drug 2 is that bound to the cell and intracellular membranes.

Pharmacokinetics and Metabolism in Drug Design.
Dennis A. Smith, Han van de Waterbeemd, Don K. Walker (Eds.)
Copyright © 2006 WILEY-VCH Verlag GmbH & Co. KGaA, Weinheim
ISBN: 3-527-31368-0

The overall amount of drug present in a tissue is determined by the amount that is bound either to intracellular proteins or, as discussed below, to the actual cell membranes themselves. Albumin is present in many tissues and organs and is available to bind drugs. Other intracellular proteins that can bind drugs include ligandin, present in liver, kidney and intestine, myosin and actin in muscular tissue, melanin in pigmented tissue, particularly the eye. Normally, as previously discussed, the free drug is that which determines the pharmacological activity. Note also from before that the concentration of free drug in the circulation depends at steady state on free drug clearance and not the extent of plasma protein or even blood binding. In certain instances, as will be discussed later, certain toxicities can derive directly due to membrane interactions (disruption, phospholipidosis, etc.). Key factors in crossing the membranes of cells are lipophilicity, as defined by the partition coefficient, hydrogen-bonding capacity [1], and molecular size [2]. For simple small molecules with a minimum of nitrogen or oxygen containing functions, a positive log D value is a good indicator of ability to cross the membrane. For more complex molecules, size and H-bonding capacity become important.

4.2
Brain Penetration

The work of Young and colleagues [1] provides a classic example of the role of increased H-bonding potential in preventing access to the CNS (crossing capillary and astrocyte cell membranes (Fig. 4.2)). In this example Δlog P provided a measure of H-bonding potential.

Much of the data produced in studies such as this measured the partitioning of drugs into whole brain from blood or plasma. The importance of lipophilicity in brain distribution has therefore been highlighted in many reviews [3, 4]. However,

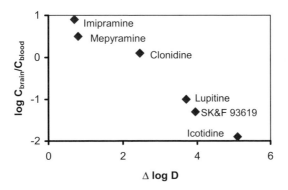

Fig. 4.2 Penetration of anti-histamine compounds into the CNS correlated with Δlog P (log P cyclohexane – log P octanol) as a measure of hydrogen-bonding potential.

the majority of these have concentrated on total drug concentrations, which, given the lipid nature of brain tissue, overemphasises the accumulation of lipophilic drugs.

Whilst giving some ideas of the penetration into the brain, such data are limited in understanding the CNS activity of drugs. Whole-brain partitioning actually represents partitioning into the lipid of the brain, and not actually access to drug receptors. For instance, desipramine partitions into the brain and is distributed unevenly [5]. The distribution corresponds to lipid content of the brain regions and not to specific desipramine binding sites. Thus correlations such as above are correlating the partitioning of the drug into a lipid against the partitioning of the drug into a model lipid. For receptors such as 7TMs ECF concentrations determine activity. The ECF can be considered the aqueous phase of the CNS. Cerebrospinal fluid (CSF) concentrations can be taken as a reasonable guide of ECF concentrations. The apparent dramatic differences in brain distribution described for total brain, as shown above (3–4 orders of magnitude), collapse to a small ratio when free (unbound) concentration of drug in plasma is compared to CSF concentration. Whole brain/blood partitioning reflects nothing but an inert partitioning process of drug into lipid material.

The lack of information conveyed by total brain concentration is indicated by studies on KA-672 [6], a lipophilic benzopyranone acetylchoinesterase inhibitor. The compound achieved total brain concentrations $0.39\,\mu M$ at a dose of $1\,mg\,kg^{-1}$, equivalent to the IC_{50} determined *in vitro* ($0.36\,\mu M$). Doses up to $10\,mg\,kg^{-1}$ were without pharmacological effect. Analysis of CSF indicated concentrations of the compound were below $0.01\,M$ readily explaining the lack of activity. These low concentrations are due presumably from high (unbound) free drug clearance and resultant low concentrations of free drug in the plasma (and CSF).

Free unbound drug partitioning actually reflects the drug reaching the receptor and pharmacological effect. Unless active transport systems are invoked the maximum CSF to plasma partition coefficient is one. This should be contrasted to the 100 or 1000-fold affinity of total brain compared to blood or plasma. The minimum partitioning based on a limited data set appears to be 0.1. Figure 4.3 compares lipophilicity (log D) to a series of diverse compounds that illustrate the limited range of partitioning. It should be noted that the term log D is not a perfect descriptor and some of the measures which incorporate size and hydrogen bonding may be better. Clearly though, the CNS is more permeable than imagined, allowing drugs like sulpiride (Fig. 4.3) to be used for CNS applications.

The use of microdialysis has enabled unbound drug concentrations to be determined in ECF, providing another measurement of penetration across the blood-brain barrier and one more closely related to activity. A review of data obtained by microdialysis [7] found free drug exposure in the brain is equal to or less than free drug concentration in plasma or blood, with ratios ranging from 4% for the most polar compound (atenolol) to unity for lipophilic compounds (e.g. carbamazepine). This largely supports the similar conclusions from the CSF data shown above. This relationship is illustrated in Fig. 4.4.

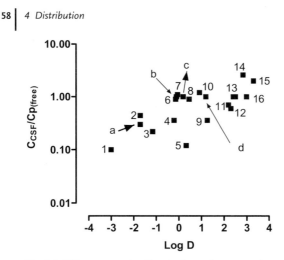

Fig. 4.3 CSF concentration/free (unbound) plasma concentration ratios for neutral and basic drugs: ritropirronium (1), atenolol (2), sulpiride (3), morphine (4), cimetidine (5), metoprolol (6), atropine (7), tacrine (8), digoxin (9), propranolol (10), carbamazepine (11), ondansetron (12), diazepam (13), imipramine (14), digitonin (15), chlorpromazine (16), and acidic drugs, salicylic acid (a), ketoprofen (b), oxyphenbutazone (c), and indomethacin (d) compared to log *D*.

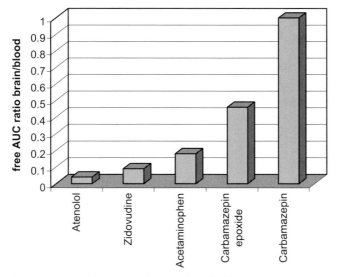

Fig. 4.4 Relationship between lipophilicity and CNS penetration expressed as free drug AUC ratio in brain to blood [16].

Somewhat surprisingly, microdialysis has also revealed that the time to maximum concentration (T_{max}) within the CNS is close to the T_{max} value in blood or plasma, irrespective of lipophilicity. For example, the CNS T_{max} for atenolol (log $D_{7.4} = -1.8$) occurs at two minutes in rats after intravenous administration [8]. In addition, the rate of elimination (half-life) of atenolol and other polar agents from the CNS is similar to that in plasma or blood. The implication of these data is that poorly permeable drugs do not take longer to reach equilibrium with CNS tissue than more lipophilic agents as might be assumed. To explain these observations, it has been postulated that non-passive transport (i.e. active) processes play a role in determining CNS exposure [7].

The fact that hydrophilic compounds have ready access to the CNS, albeit up to tenfold lower than lipophilic compounds, is not generally appreciated. In the design of drugs selectivity over the CNS effects has sometimes relied on making compounds hydrophilic. Clearly this will give some selectivity (up to tenfold), but this may not be enough. For instance β-adrenoceptor antagonists are known to cause sleep disorders. In four drugs studied the effects were lowest with atenolol (log $D = -1.6$), intermediate with metoprolol (log $D = -0.1$), and highest with pindolol (log $D = -0.1$) and propranolol (log $D = 1.2$). This was correlated with the total amount present in brain tissue [9], which related to the log D values. Further analysis of the data [10] using CSF data and receptor affinity to calculate receptor occupancy demonstrated that there was high occupation of the β_1 central receptor for all drugs. Propranolol showed a low occupancy, possibly because the active 4-hydroxy metabolite is not included in the calculation. In contrast, occupation of the β_2 central receptor correlated well with sleep disturbances. The incidence of sleep disturbances is therefore not about penetration into the CNS but the β_1/β_2 selectivity of the compounds (atenolol > metoprolol > pindolol = propranolol). The relative receptor occupancies are illustrated in Fig. 4.5.

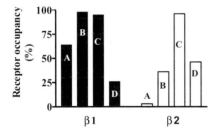
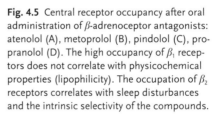

Fig. 4.5 Central receptor occupancy after oral administration of β-adrenoceptor antagonists: atenolol (A), metoprolol (B), pindolol (C), propranolol (D). The high occupancy of β_1 receptors does not correlate with physicochemical properties (lipophilicity). The occupation of β_2 receptors correlates with sleep disturbances and the intrinsic selectivity of the compounds.

For a small drug molecule, penetration to the target may often be easier to achieve than duration of action. Assuming duration of action is linked to drug half-life, then distribution as outlined below can be an important factor.

4.3
Volume of Distribution and Duration

The volume of distribution of a drug molecule is, as described previously, a theoretical number that assumes the drug is at equal concentration in the tissue to that in the circulation and represents what volume (or mass) of tissue is required to give that concentration. Volume of distribution, therefore, provides a term that partially reflects tissue affinity. However, it is important to remember that affinity may vary between different tissues and a moderate volume of distribution may reflect moderate concentrations in many tissues or high concentrations in a few. For the illustration of how the manipulation of distribution affects systemic concentration the examples will use free volume rather than total, although either could equally apply.

Taking the simplest case of neutral drugs, where increasing log $D_{7.4}$ reflects increased binding to constituents of blood and cells and increased partitioning of drugs into membranes, there is a trend for increasing volume of distribution with increasing lipophilicity (Fig. 4.6). In this case, for uncharged neutral molecules, there are no additional ionic interactions with tissue constituents. In most cases, the volume of distribution is highest for basic drugs ionised at physiological pH, due to ion-pair interactions between the basic centre and the charged acidic head groups of phospholipid membranes as described previously.

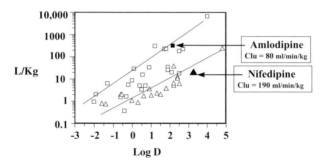

Fig. 4.6 Free (unbound) volumes of distribution of neutral (triangles) and basic (squares) drugs, also indicating amlodipine and nifedipine together with their free (unbound) clearance value (Cl_u).

This ion pairing for basic drugs means high affinity and also that the ionised fraction of the drug is the predominant form within the membrane. This is particularly important, since most alkylamines have pK_a values in the range 8-10 and are, thus, predominantly ionised at physiological pH. The increase in volume for basic drugs is also illustrated in Fig. 4.6.

The importance of volume of distribution is in influencing the duration of drug effect. Since half-life ($0.693/k_{el}$, where k_{el} is the elimination rate constant) is determined by the volume of distribution and the clearance ($Cl_u = V_{d(f)} \times k_{el}$), manipulation of volume is an important tool for changing duration of action. Here the small amount of drug in the circulation is important, since this is the compound actually passing through and hence available to the organs of clearance (liver and kidney). Incorporation of a basic centre into a neutral molecule is therefore a method of increasing the volume of distribution of a compound. An example of this is the discovery of the series of drugs based on rifamycin SV (Fig. 4.7). This

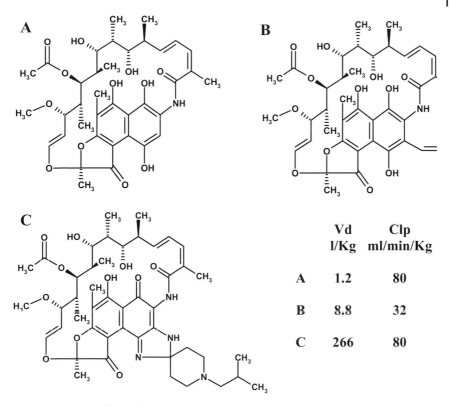

Fig. 4.7 Structures of (A) rifamycin, (B) rifampicin and (C) rifabutin, together with their pharmacokinetic properties. Volume of distribution (V_d) and plasma clearance (Cl_p) are for free unbound drug.

compound was one of the first drugs with high activity against *Mycobacterium tuberculosis*. Its clinical performance [11], however, was disappointing due to poor oral absorption (dissolution) and very short duration ascribed at the time to rapid biliary elimination (clearance).

Many different analogues were produced, including introduction of basic functions with a goal of increased potency, solubility, and reduction in clearance. Rifampicin is a methyl-piperazinyl amino methyl derivative [12] with much better duration and a successful drug. The basic functionality however does not alter clearance but increases volume substantially (Fig. 4.7). Duration is enhanced further [12] by the more basic spiropiperidyl analogue, rifabutin (Fig. 4.7). Again the desirable pharmacokinetic (and pharmacodynamic) properties are due to effects on volume of distribution rather than effects on clearance.

This strategy of modification of a neutral molecule by addition of basic functionality was employed in the discovery of the dihydropyridine calcium channel blocker, amlodipine. The long plasma elimination half-life (35 hours) of amlodipine (Fig. 4.8) is due, in large part, to its basicity and resultant high volume of distribution [13].

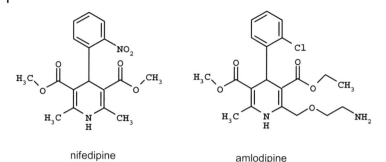

nifedipine   amlodipine

Fig. 4.8 Structures of the dihydropyridine calcium channel blockers, nifedipine (neutral) and amlodipine (basic).

These pharmacokinetic parameters are unique among dihydropyridine calcium channel blockers and allow once a day dosing of amlodipine, without the need for sustained release technology. The large volume of distribution is achieved despite the moderate lipophilicity of amlodipine and can be compared to the prototype dihydropyridine drug, nifedipine, which is of similar lipophilicity but neutral (Fig. 4.8). Notably, these changes in structure do not trigger a large change in clearance. The high tissue distribution of amlodipine is unique amongst dihydropyridine drugs, and has been ascribed to a specific ionic interaction between the protonated amino function and the charged anionic oxygen of the phosphate headgroups present in the phospholipid membranes [14] (see Chapter 1 on physicochemistry).

Another basic drug where minor structural modification results in a dramatic increase in volume of distribution is the macrolide antibiotic, azithromycin. The traditional agent in this class is erythromycin, which contains one basic nitrogen, in the sugar sidechain.

Introduction of a second basic centre into the macrolide aglycone ring in azithromycin increases the free (unbound) volume of distribution from 4.8 L kg^{-1} to 62 L kg^{-1} (Fig. 4.9). Free (unbound) clearance of the two compounds is also changed from 55 mL per min per kg for erythromycin to 18 mL per min per kg for azithromycin. The apparent plasma elimination half-life is, therefore, increased from 3 to 48 hours. One consequence of the high tissue distribution of azithromycin is that the plasma or blood concentrations do not reflect tissue levels, which may be ten to 100-fold higher, compared to only 0.5 to fivefold higher for erythromycin. Azithromycin readily enters macrophages and leukocytes and is, therefore, particularly beneficial against intracellular pathogens. Elimination of azithromycin is also prolonged with reported tissue half-life values of up to 77 hours [15]. Overall, the pharmacokinetic properties of azithromycin provide adequate tissue concentrations on a once-daily dosing regimen and provide wide therapeutic applications. The high and prolonged tissue concentrations of azithromycin achieved provide a long duration of action. Only three to five day courses of treatment are, therefore, required, hence improving patient compliance to complete the course and reducing development of resistance [15].

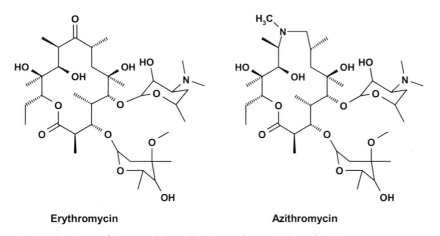

Erythromycin   **Azithromycin**

Fig. 4.9 Structures of the macrolide antibiotics, erythromycin (monobasic) and azithromycin (dibasic).

A similar example to azithromycin, but in a small molecule series is pholcodine (Fig. 4.10), where a basic morpholino side chain replaces the methyl group of codeine. Unbound clearance is essentially similar (10 mL per min per kg) but the free unbound volume is increased approximately tenfold (4 to 40 L kg^{-1}) with a corresponding increase in half-life (3 to 37 hours) [16].

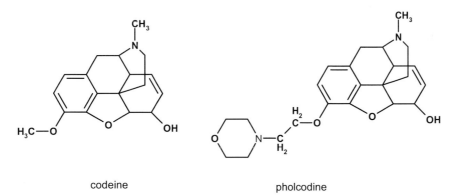

codeine   pholcodine

Fig. 4.10 Structures of codeine (monobasic) and pholcodine (dibasic).

High accumulation of drug in tissues has also been implicated in the seven times longer elimination half-life of the dibasic anti-arrhythmic, disobutamide (Fig. 4.11), compared to the monobasic agents, disopyramide. The elimination half life of disobutamide is 54 hours compared to approximately seven hours for disopyramide.

Disobutamide has been shown to accumulate extensively in tissues in contrast to disopyramide [17].

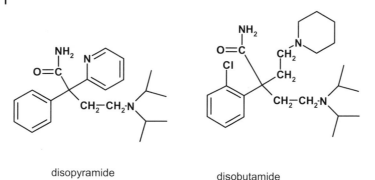

disopyramide   disobutamide

Fig. 4.11 Structures of the monobasic anti-arrhythmic disopyramide and the dibasic analogue disobutamide.

It is important to note that in these latter two examples, the high tissue affinity of the well-tolerated, anti-infective azithromycin is viewed as a pharmacokinetic advantage, while similar high tissue affinity is viewed as disadvantageous for the low safety margin, anti-arrhythmic, disobutamide. Obviously, different therapeutic areas impose different restrictions on the ideal pharmacokinetic profile for management of each condition. Hence, careful consideration should be paid to this at an early stage in drug discovery programmes.

4.4
Distribution and T_{max}

It has been postulated that high tissue distribution of drugs can lead to a delayed T_{max} (time to maximum plasma concentration) after oral administration. Amlodipine (Fig. 4.5), has a typical T_{max} value of six to nine hours following an oral dose. Given the excellent physicochemical properties (moderately lipophilic and good solubility) of this molecule, slow absorption across the membranes of the gastrointestinal tract is unlikely. In addition, the compound appears to be more rapidly absorbed in patients with hepatic impairment with a mean T_{max} value of 3.8 versus 6.8 hours [18]. The apparent slow absorption has been attributed to the considerable partitioning of drugs like amlodipine into the initial tissue beds encountered followed by a slower redistribution. After oral dosing the major tissue bed is the liver. The intrinsic high tissue distribution of amlodipine is reflected in a volume of distribution of 21 L kg^{-1} [19]. Amlodipine, which is a relatively low clearance compound, is thus taken up extensively into the liver and then slowly redistributes back out, thus delaying the time to the maximum observed concentration in the systemic circulation (T_{max}). In the patients with hepatic impairment, the presence of hepatic shunts (blood vessels bypassing the liver) decreases the exposure of the compound to liver tissue and hence reduces T_{max}. Studies with isolated rat livers indicated that the apparent volume of distribution of the liver exceeded 100 mL g^{-1} tissue demonstrating very high affinity for this tissue [20].

This postulated phenomenon can have the beneficial effect of reducing the likelihood of systemic side effects by effectively buffering the rate at which drugs enter the systemic circulation and hence reducing peak to trough variations in concentration. Conversely, high affinity for liver tissue may increase exposure to the enzymes of clearance and may therefore attenuate the first-pass extraction of drugs.

References

1 Young, R.C., Mitchell, R.C., Brown, T.H., Ganellin, C.R., Griffiths, R., Jones, M., Rana, K.K., Saunders, D., Smith, I.R., Sore, N.E., Wilks, T.J. **1988**, *J. Med. Chem.* 31, 656–671.

2 Van de Waterbeemd, H., Camenisch, G., Folkers, G., Chrétien, J.R., Raevsky, O.A. **1998**, *J. Drug Target.* 6, 151–165.

3 Brodie, B.B., Kurz, H., Schanker, L.S. **1960**, *J. Pharmacol. Exp. Ther.* 130, 20–25.

4 Hansch, C., Bjorkroth, J.P., Leo, A. **1987**, *J. Pharm. Sci.* 76, 663–687.

5 Wladyslaw, D., Leokadia, D., Lucyna, J., Halina, N., Miroslawa, M. **1991**, *J. Pharm. Pharmacol.* 43, 31–35.

6 Hilgert, M., Noldner, M., Chatterjee, S.S., Klein, J. **1999**, *J. Neurosci. Lett.* 263, 193–196.

7 Hammarlund-Udenaes, M., Paalzow, L.K., De Lange, E.C.M. **1997**, *Pharm. Res.* 14, 128–134.

8 De Lange, E.C.M., Danhof, M., deBoer, A.G., Breimer, D.D. **1994**, *Brain Res.* 666, 1–8.

9 McAinsh, J., Cruickshank, J.M. **1990**, *Pharmac. Therap.* 46, 163–197.

10 Yamada, Y., Shibuya, F., Hamada, J., Shawada, Y., Iga, T. **1995**, *J. Pharmacokinet. Biopharm.* 23, 131–145.

11 Bergamini, N., Fowst, G. **1965**, *Arzneimittel-Forschung* 15, 951–1002.

12 Benet, L.Z., Oie, S., Schwartz, J.B. **1995**, Design and optimization of dosage regimens; pharmacokinetic data, in *Goodman and Gillman's The Pharmacological Basis for Therapeutics*, McGraw-Hill, New York, (pp.) 1707–1792.

13 Smith, D.A., Jones, B.C., Walker, D.K. **1996**, *Med. Res. Revs.* 16, 243–266.

14 Mason, R.P., Rhodes, D.G., Herbette, L.G. **1991**, *J. Med. Chem.* 34, 869–877.

15 Foulds, G., Shepard, R.M., Johnson, R.B. **1990**, *J. Antimicrob. Chemother.* 25, Suppl. A, 73–82.

16 Fowle, W.A., Butz, A.S.E., Jones, E.C., Waetherly, B.C., Welch, R.M., Posner, J. **1986**, *Br. J. Clin. Pharmacol.* 22, 61–71.

17 Cook, C.S., McDonald, S.J., Karim, A. **1993**, *Xenobiotica* 23, 1299–1309.

18 Humphrey, M.J., Smith, D.A. **1992**, *Br. J. Clin. Pharmacol.* 33, 219P.

19 Faulkner, J.K., McGibney, D., Chasseaud, L.F., Perry, J.L., Taylor, I.W. **1986**, *Br. J. Clin. Pharmacol.* 22, 21–25.

20 Walker, D.K., Humphrey, M.J., Smith, D.A. **1994**, *Xenobiotica* 24, 243–250.

5
Clearance

5.1
The Clearance Processes

Clearance of drug normally occurs from the liver and kidneys and it is an important assumption that only the free (i.e. not protein bound) drug is available for clearance. A diagram of the interaction of the major clearance processes is shown in Fig. 5.1.

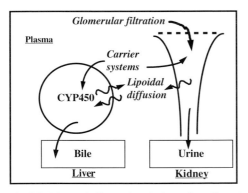

Fig. 5.1 Schematic illustrating the interplay of hepatic and renal clearance processes.

All compounds are filtered by the glomerulus (Chapter 6) but lipophilic compounds are reabsorbed, as they are readily able to permeate the lipid membranes and thus return to the systemic circulation. Drugs are normally lipophilic in nature and lipophilicity is a key factor in determining the intrinsic affinity of a drug for its target or other proteins (such as CYP450, see Section 7.2.3) as well as its absorbability (see Section 3.3). Lipophilicity therefore also governs the requirement of a drug to be metabolised to substances that can be voided in the urine. The liver is the principal site of metabolism. Figure 5.2 illustrates the importance of the three primary routes of clearance when the top 200 drugs, as judged by prescriptions filled, are considered and demonstrates the importance of metabolism.

Pharmacokinetics and Metabolism in Drug Design.
Dennis A. Smith, Han van de Waterbeemd, Don K. Walker (Eds.)
Copyright © 2006 WILEY-VCH Verlag GmbH & Co. KGaA, Weinheim
ISBN: 3-527-31368-0

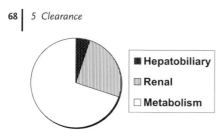

Fig. 5.2 Primary clearance route of the top 200 drugs as judged
on a prescription basis and the importance of metabolism.

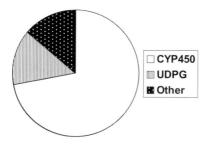

Fig. 5.3 The enzyme responsible for the primary metabolic
clearance route (shown in Fig. 5.2) of the top 200 drugs as judged
on a prescription basis and the importance of CYP450.

Further consideration of which enzymes are involved is shown in Fig. 5.3 and
illustrates that cytochrome P450s (CYP450) and uridine diphosphate glucuronyl
transferases (UDPGTs) are the most important, with the CYPs predominant.

5.2
Role of Transport Proteins in Drug Clearance

For hepatic clearance, passive diffusion through the lipid core of the hepatocyte
membranes (available only to lipophilic drugs) is augmented by sinusoidal carrier
systems, particularly for ionised molecules (either anionic or cationic) of molecular weights above 400. The presence of these carrier systems provides access to
the interior of the hepatocyte to drugs with a wide range of physicochemical properties, ranging from hydrophilic to lipophilic. A schematic illustrating the role of
these transport systems both into the liver and out of the liver is shown in Fig.
5.4. The transporters exist on the sinusoid face to remove drugs from the blood
and transport them into the interior of the hepatocyte [1].

Likewise a different family of transporters exists on the canalicular face to transport drugs or their metabolites into bile. This complex system was originally
termed biliary clearance but it is really two separate processes, hepatic uptake and
biliary excretion. With small sized lipophilic drugs that readily traverse membranes, hepatic uptake is probably not a major factor, even if compounds are sub-

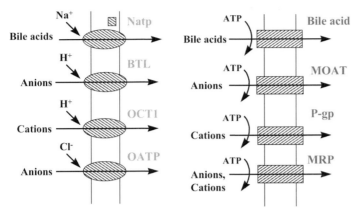

Fig. 5.4 Schematic showing key sinusoidal and canalicular transport proteins and their substrate characteristics.

strates, rapid redistribution across the membrane can occur. With higher molecular weight compounds (molecular weight greater than about 500) and those containing considerable H-bonding functionality (i.e. those that do not readily cross membranes) hepatic uptake can become the key clearance process, even if metabolism occurs subsequent to this. Figure 5.5 shows the structure of two combined thromboxane synthase inhibitors, thromboxane A_2 receptor antagonists (TxSI/ TxRAs). Both compounds show high hepatic extraction ($E = 0.9$) in the isolated perfused rat liver [2].

Compound A appears mainly as unchanged drug in the bile whereas compound B appears partly as metabolites. Administration of ketoconazole, a potent cytochrome P450 inhibitor, to the preparation dramatically decreases the metabolism of B and the compound appears mainly as unchanged material in the bile. Despite the inhibition of metabolism, hepatic extraction remains high (0.9). This indicates that clearance is dependent on hepatic uptake, via a transporter system, for removal of the compounds from the circulation. Metabolism of compound B

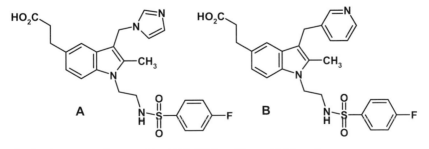

Fig. 5.5 Structures of two combined TxSI/TxRAs subject to high hepatic extraction by sinusoidal transport systems.

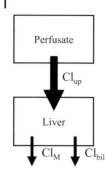

Fig. 5.6 Model for the hepatic processes involved in the clearance of the combined TxSI/TxRAs (see Fig. 5.5). The clearance by hepatic uptake (Cl_{up}) is the rate-determining step in the removal of compound from the perfusate. Compounds accumulate within the liver and are subsequently cleared by biliary (Cl_{bil}) or metabolic clearance (Cl_M) (modified from [2]).

is a process that occurs subsequent to this rate-determining step and does not influence overall clearance. This model for the various processes involved in the clearance of these compounds is illustrated in Fig. 5.6.

The affinity of compounds for the various transporter proteins vary, but charge, molecular weight and additional H-bonding functionality seem to be particularly important.

Lipophilic drugs are metabolised by intracellular membrane bound enzyme systems (e.g. cytochrome P450s and glucuronyl transferases) to more water soluble derivatives. The active sites of the major forms of the cytochrome P450 superfamily rely heavily on hydrophobic interactions with their substrates, although ion-pair and hydrogen-bonding interactions also occur. Exit from the hepatocyte may be by simple passive diffusion back into the plasma or as outlined above via canalicular active transport systems, which excrete drugs and their metabolites, again with wide ranging physicochemical properties, into the bile.

5.3
Interplay Between Metabolic and Renal Clearance

Small molecules, with relatively low molecular weight, will appear in the urine due to glomerular filtration. The secretion of drugs into the urine can also occur through tubular carrier systems similar to those present on the sinusoid face of the hepatocyte. For instance, of the carriers illustrated in Fig. 5.4, Natp, OATP and OCT1 are also present in the kidney. In addition another organic cation transporter, OCT2, is also present. There is also a vast difference in the volume of fluid formed at the glomerulus each minute and the amount that arrives during the same period at the collecting tubule. The aqueous concentration processes that occur in the kidney mean that for drugs capable of travelling through the lipid core of the tubule membrane, significant reabsorption back into the plasma will occur. This process has the end result of only hydrophilic molecules being voided in the urine to any substantial degree. This interaction between metabolism and renal clearance can be illustrated by following the fate of the cholinesterase inhibitor SM-10888 [3]. A number of metabolism processes occur on the lipophilic

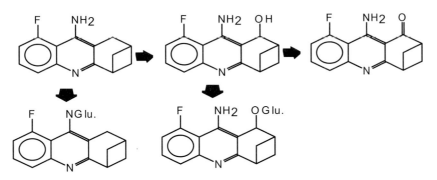

Fig. 5.7 Metabolism of SM-10888, involving phase I and phase II metabolic processes.

parent molecule involving phase I oxidation and phase II conjugation reactions. Some of these processes occur sequentially as illustrated in Fig. 5.7.

5.4
Role of Lipophilicity in Drug Clearance

Most of these steps result in a reduction in lipophilicity compared to the parent molecule. These reductions in lipophilicity lead to an increased renal clearance and effectively permit the voiding of the dose from the body as illustrated in Fig. 5.8.

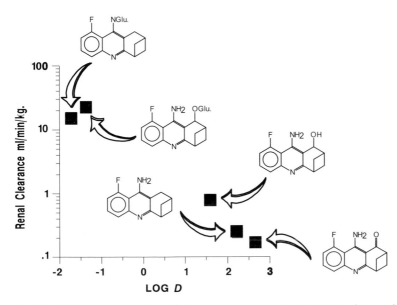

Fig. 5.8 Relationship between lipophilicity and renal clearance for SM 10888 and its metabolites.

This demonstrates the interaction between metabolic and renal clearance. Assuming that SM-10888 is the only pharmacologically active moiety, these processes govern the clearance of active drug and hence determine the required dose. In fact, only the formation of the N-glucuronide and the benzylic hydroxyl metabolites are of prime concern to the medicinal chemist. These represent the primary clearance routes of the compound and hence govern the rate of clearance, and ultimately the dosage regimen needed to obtain a particular plasma concentration of the active compound, SM-10888 in this example.

The reduction in lipophilicity normally observed with metabolism means that most often metabolites are less intrinsically active than the parent. When active, metabolites usually possess similar pharmacology to the parent rather than introduce novel *de novo* pharmacology. In many drugs (notably those acting on aminergic receptors and transporters), the presence of a tertiary amine function leads to metabolism along a sequential pathway of N-dealkylation reactions through the secondary amine to the primary amine (see Section 7.2.3). Due to the increased metabolic stability of these metabolites (ease of electron abstraction, see Section 7.2.3) it is often found that they have greater duration in the circulation than the parent and thus exert a longer lasting effect if active. Moreover, more accumulation of the metabolite will occur leading to a greater influence of activity with repeated dosing of the parent drug. Due to this common finding the appropriate metabolites should always be synthesised and tested for activity, and if active to within five to tenfold of parent, be included in pre-clinical and clinical assessment to understand their role in the pharmacodynamics of the drug.

Rather than looking at a metabolism pathway, similar models for the control of the mechanism of clearance by lipophilicity are demonstrated by considering drugs in general. Figure 5.9 illustrates free drug renal and metabolic clearance for a series of neutral compounds drawn from the literature [4].

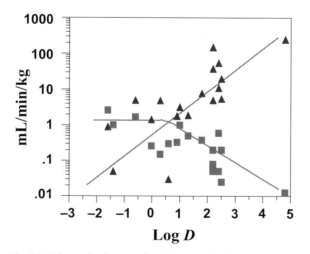

Fig. 5.9 Relationship between lipophilicity and unbound renal (squares) and metabolic clearance (triangles) for a range of neutral drugs in man.

For hydrophilic drugs (log $D_{7.4}$ below zero) renal clearance is the predominant mechanism. For drugs with log $D_{7.4}$ values above zero, renal clearance decreases with lipophilicity. In contrast to renal clearance, metabolic clearance increases with increasing log D and this becomes the major clearance route of lipophilic compounds. Noticeably, considering the logarithmic scale in Fig. 5.9, overall clearance decreases with decreasing lipophilicity. The lowest clearances, by the combined renal and metabolic processes, are observed below log $D_{7.4}$ values of zero, where metabolic clearance is negligible. This apparent advantage needs to be offset against the disadvantages of reliance on gastrointestinal absorption via the aqueous pore pathway that will tend to predominate for hydrophilic compounds. Moreover the actual potency of the compound is also normally affected by lipophilicity with potency tending to increase with increasing lipophilicity [5]. Furthermore, as shown previously, volume of distribution also increases with increasing lipophilicity and hence tends to increase the elimination half-life ($t_{1/2} = 0.693 \times V_d/Cl$). Figure 5.10 illustrates this interdependency and highlights the importance of a combined consideration of the properties of absorption (Chapter 3), distribution (Chapter 4) and clearance (this chapter) together with pharmacology. Consideration of these processes in isolation from each other runs the substantial risk that concomitant effects on the other processes will be overlooked. These concepts have been previously mentioned in part: the purpose here is to highlight them as they are fundamental to drug design. The use of unbound free drug concentration rather than total drug allows for a numerical rather than conceptual description (see Section 2.8). Following absorption, the dose and duration of effect of a compound largely depend on the rate of metabolism or plasma clearance of a compound, its volume of distribution and its intrinsic potency. These are the properties that describe drug-like behaviour.

β-adrenergic antagonists and calcium channel antagonists provide compelling examples of the interplay between these factors, although other drug classes could have been chosen [6, 7, 8].

Considering first the β-adrenergic antagonists: the marketed compounds have an intrinsic *in vitro* potency as measured by pA_2 values ranging from 6.5 to 8.8

The triad of systemic effect

Intrinsic Potency

Absorption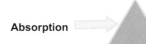

Clearance (*Cl*)   **Distribution (V_d)**

$Cl = V_d \times kel$ where $kel = 0.693/t_{1/2}$

Fig. 5.10 The triad of systemic effect. The unbound free clearance, the unbound free volume and the intrinsic potency govern dose size and duration once absorption is taken into account.

(atenolol and betaxolol), respectively. Despite the magnitude of these differences the daily dose of most of these agents is in the range of 25–100 mg.

Yamada [6] has illustrated how the pharmacokinetics of the β-adrenergic antagonists combined with daily dose and affinity yield the same degree of receptor occupancy (80%) and hence efficacy (see Section 2.9). Another feature of the diversity of compounds is their range of lipophilicity, as measured by log $D_{7.4}$ or log P, which spans four log units (see Section 1.2). Since lipophilicity is a key parameter in determining affinity for receptors (potency), enzymes (clearance), tissues and membranes (volume) and permeability (tubular reabsorption), it is illuminating to examine the various trends in these parameters that changes in lipophilicity invoke. This range in physicochemical characteristics, in particular lipophilicity, of this class of agent has been widely recognised and the impact of lipophilicity on the processes of absorption [9], distribution [10] and route [11] and rate [12] of clearance has been previously considered.

Figure 5.11 illustrates the structures of ten clinically used β-adrenoceptor antagonists. In terms of structural features and pharmacological activity, all contain the same aryloxy-propan-2-ol amino unit as a basic pharmacophore. The aryl unit shows different substituent positions, the para-position substituents giving cardioselectivity ($β_1/β_2$ specificity, e.g. atenolol). Amino substitution is either isopropyl or tertiary butyl, except for carvedilol which combines α and β-adrenoceptor antagonism.

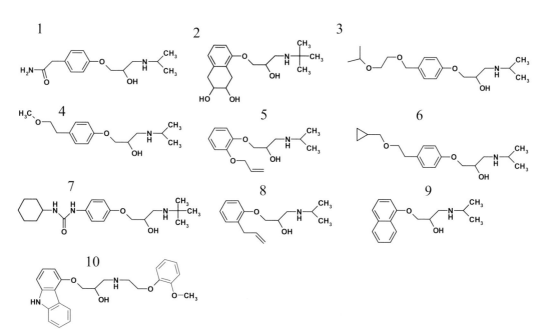

Fig. 5.11 Structures of atenolol (1), nadolol (2), bisoprolol (3), metoprolol (4), oxprenolol (5), betaxolol (6), talinolol (7), alprenolol (8), propranolol (9), carvedilol (10).

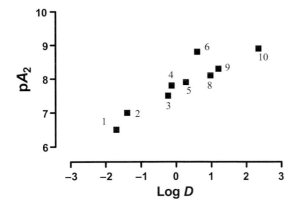

Fig. 5.12 Correlation of lipophilicity (log $D_{7.4}$) with *in vitro* potency (pA$_2$).

Figure 5.12 illustrates the potency of the members of this series of compounds against the β_1 receptor, expressed as a pA$_2$ value. The potency shows a marked correlation with lipophilicity with a 300-fold increase in potency (based on pA$_2$ values) associated with a 10 000-fold increase in lipophilicity (D or P). Such changes can be simply rationalised considering the features of the natural agonists (e.g. adrenaline) and the key binding interactions, which the aryloxy-propan-2-ol amino unit fulfils. Any increase in potency is likely to come from more non-specific lipophilic interactions.

Figure 5.13 shows the relationship between unbound volume and lipophilicity. The major component of volume of distribution is the affinity for the membranes of cells. This affinity is derived from two physiochemical properties: the compounds intrinsic lipophilicity and its basicity. Membranes are comprised of phospholipids with charged head groups, some acidic, and lipid tails organised as a bilayer to form a lipid interior. Lipophilicity determines the compounds ability to interact with the lipid core of the membrane, whilst the basic nitrogen group

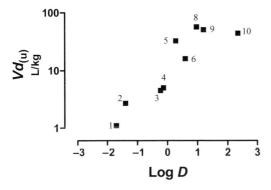

Fig. 5.13 Correlation of lipophilicity (log $D_{7.4}$) with unbound (free) volume of distribution (V_{du}).

allows ion-pair interactions with the ionised head groups. Since the compounds all possess a similar basic centre (pK_a 9.4), their lipophilicity is the predominant driving force in determining volume. The strong correlation between unbound (free) volume and lipophilicity is in keeping with these interactions.

Figure 5.14 contrasts the unbound intrinsic clearance (Cl_{iu}) and unbound renal clearance (Cl_{Ru}) with lipophilicity for these agents. Unbound renal clearance is approximately constant over the range illustrated (log $D_{7.4}$ –2 to +1), however, it probably declines with compounds of higher lipophilicity (see Chapter 6). The amount excreted in urine (as a proportion of the administered dose) decreases dramatically with lipophilicity due to the increased importance of metabolic clearance, making calculations unreliable for the more lipophilic examples. Metabolic clearance (as unbound intrinsic clearance) is described in detail across the whole lipophilicity range (log $D_{7.4}$ –2 to +2.5). The intrinsic affinity of the enzymes of clearance exhibits an almost stochastic relationship with the lipophilicity of the compounds. This relationship between lipophilicity and clearance is very important as a fundamental principal (albeit with caveats).

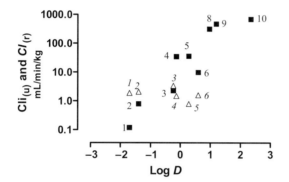

Fig. 5.14 Correlation of lipophilicity (log $D_{7.4}$) with unbound (free) hepatic intrinsic clearance (Cl_{iu}: filled squares) and unbound (free) renal clearance (Cl_{Ru}: open triangles).

Figure 5.15 illustrates the rate of metabolism obtained from disappearance half-life estimations *in vitro* using human liver microsomes for several β-adrenoceptor antagonists. There is in general a good relationship with lipophilicity, but compound 6 (betaxolol) appears to be more stable. This is emphasised in the insert plot showing a linear rate scale.

Rate of metabolism is a function of chemical lability and the ability to enter and leave the active site of the enzyme. Clearly actual functionality must play a role (one of the caveats referred to above in the lipophilicity/clearance relationship), rather than just the lipophilicity of the substituent. Comparison can be made between compound 4 (metoprolol) and compound 6 (betaxolol). Metoprolol has an ethoxymethyl para-substituent that renders the compound liable to metabolism at both the benzylic and methyl position. In contrast betoxolol has an ethyoxymethyl

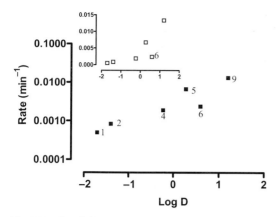

Fig. 5.15 Plot of elimination rate constant for the *in vitro* metabolism of selected *β*-adrenoceptor antagonists against lipophilicity.

cyclopropyl substituent that is less prone to metabolism (see Section 7.2.1). Whilst these differences are very important the overall trend is that much of the chemistry around the basic aryloxy-propan-2-ol amino unit has the effect of changing potency and key pharmacokinetic properties in a compensating manner. The affinity of fluorinated analogues of propranolol for the drug metabolising enzyme CYP1A2 has been shown to be altered by changes in pK_a [13]. Reducing the amine pK_a by additional substitution of fluoro or alkyl substituents in the 1'-position of the N-isopropyl group was associated with an increase in lipophilicity (log $D_{7.4}$). The increased lipid partitioning of the analogues resulted in increased affinity for CYP1A2 (lower K_m) and increased catalytic efficiency. In these examples, steric factors (e.g. size of substituent group) appear to have a greater influence on the routes of metabolism of the individual compounds.

To further emphasise the balance needed in drug design, extremes of the *β*-adrenoceptor antagonists, atenolol and propranolol [6], have been chosen (Table 5.1). These have differing physicochemical properties. Atenolol is a hydrophilic compound, shows reduced absorption, low clearance predominantly by the renal route and a moderate volume of distribution. Note that the absorption by the paracellular route (see Section 3.3) is still high, due to the small size of this class of agent. In contrast propranolol, a moderately lipophilic compound, shows high absorption, high clearance via metabolism and a large volume of distribution. Because of this balance of properties both compounds exhibit very similar elimination half-lives. These half-lives are sufficiently long for both drugs to be administered on twice daily (bd) dosage regimens due to the relatively flat dose response curves of this class of agent.

Propranolol is considerably more potent (albeit less selective) than atenolol. Thus, despite a much higher clearance than atenolol, both agents have a daily clinical dose size of around 25–100 mg.

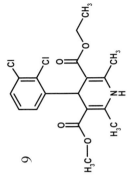

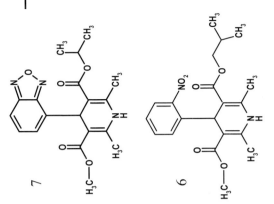

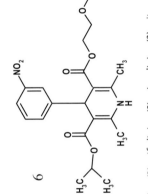

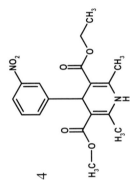

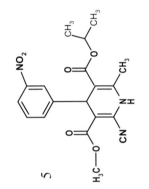

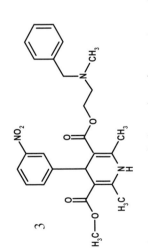

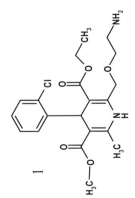

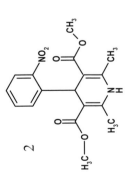

Fig. 5.16 Structures of calcium channel antagonists: amlodipine (1), nifedipine (2), nicardipine (3), nitrendipine (4), nilvaldipine (5), nimodipine (6), isradipine (7), nisoldipine (8), felodipine (9).

Tab. 5.1 Physicochemical, pharmacological and pharmacokinetic properties for atenolol and propranolol illustrating their interdependence.

	Log $D_{7.4}$	Affinity (nM)	Absorption (%)	Oral clearance (unbound) mL per min per kg	Volume of distribution (unbound) L kg^{-1}	Half-life (hours)
Atenolol	−1.9	100	50	4	0.8	3–5
Propranolol	1.1	4	100	700	51	3–5

As shown above using the example of β-adrenoceptor antagonists, increasing lipophilicity raises both V_{du} and Cl_{iu}, effectively cancelling out any changes in half-life. Moreover the daily dose size is governed by the steady state concentration of unbound drug and potency. The dihydropyridine calcium channel antagonists (Fig. 5.16) also demonstrate similar strong trends between lipophilicity and unbound intrinsic clearance (Cl_{iu}) and unbound volume (V_{du}) (Figs. 5.17 and 5.18).

The relationship for Cl_{iu} and lipophilicity is again striking (Fig. 5.17), but is perhaps unsurprising as invariably oxidation of the dihydropyridine ring, via an electron abstraction process, is the common primary clearance step. Further metabolism of the pyridine metabolite occurs on the various side chain substituents involving ester hydrolysis and alkyl hydroxylation [14]. This oxidation is conducted by CYP3A4 [15], an enzyme whose interactions are primarily lipophilic (see Section 7.2.3).

The relationship with volume and lipophilicity (Fig. 5.18) reflects the interaction with these predominantly neutral molecules (see below for ionised molecules

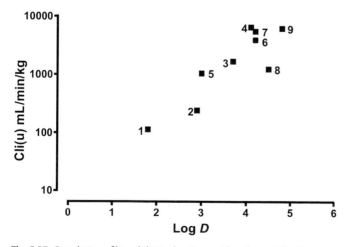

Fig. 5.17 Correlation of lipophilicity (log $D_{7.4}$) with unbound (free) hepatic intrinsic clearance (Cl_{iu}) for selected dihydropyridine calcium channel antagonists.

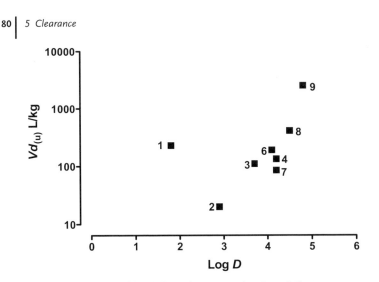

Fig. 5.18 Correlation of lipophilicity (log $D_{7.4}$) with unbound (free) volume of distribution (V_{du}) for selected dihydropyridine calcium channel antagonists. Compounds 2–9 are neutral at physiological pH, whereas amlodipine, compound 1, is basic and ionised.

such as amlodipine) and the lipid portion of biological membranes. Thus there is a high dependence on lipophilicity, also the volume/lipophilicity ratio is lower than for the basic β-adrenoceptor antagonists, referred to above, due to the absence of the ion-pair interaction.

Despite the structural diversity, in general most of the compounds have a relatively short half-life (around two to five hours). This is due to the moderate volumes of distribution and high intrinsic clearance, and their close relationship with lipophilicity. Most compounds therefore require frequent inconvenient dosage regimens. Amlodipine (compound 1), as described in Section 4.3, incorporates a basic centre and the additional interactions with charged phospholipid head groups (Fig. 5.18) gives the compound a larger volume than expected for neutral dihydropyridines.

These interrelationships illustrate why it is bad practice to optimise on only one property, such as *in vitro* potency. Invariably, this will drive the SAR towards more lipophilic compounds. In fact, better drug-like properties will not result from this strategy, due to interplay on pharmacokinetic parameters and ultimately solubility and dissolution will be adversely attenuated (Section 3.2). The anti-fungal agent fluconazole provides the classic example, where despite vastly inferior potency (MIC 3.1 mcg mL^{-1}) compared to classic anti-fungal agents such as itraconazole (MIC 0.01 mcg mL^{-1}), its pharmacokinetic advantages [16] in terms of improved solubility and absorption and reduced unbound intrinsic clearance result in a similar daily dose size of around 100 mg day^{-1} with reduced variability. Optimal properties may reside over a span of lipophilicities as illustrated by the β-adrenoceptor antagonists. However, analysis of over 200 marketed oral drugs illustrates the distribution shown in Fig. 5.19, where most drugs reside in the *middle ground* of phy-

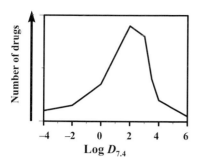

Fig. 5.19 Analysis of marketed oral drugs and their lipophilic properties.

siochemical properties with log $D_{7.4}$ values in the range zero to three. This is probably by act rather than design, but intuitively it fits with the idea of maximising oral potency, absorption and duration by balancing intrinsic potency, dissolution, membrane transfer, distribution and metabolism.

References

1 Muller, M, Jansen, P.L.M. **1997**, *Am. J. Physiol.* 272, G1285–G1303.

2 Gardner, I.B., Walker, D.K., Lennard, M.S., Smith, D.A., Tucker, G.T. **1995**, *Xenobiotica* 25, 185–197.

3 Yabuki, M., Mine, T., Iba, K., Nakatsuka, I., Yoshitake, A. **1994**, *Drug Metab. Dispos.* 22, 294–297.

4 Smith, D.A. **1997**, Physicochemical properties in drug metabolism and pharmacokinetics, in *Computer-Assisted Lead Finding and Optimisation*, Van de Waterbeemd, H., Testa, B., Folkers, G. (eds.), Wiley-VCH, Weinheim, (pp.) 265–276.

5 Lipinski, C.A., Lombardo, F., Dominy, B.W., Feeney, P.J. **1997**, *Adv. Drug Del. Rev.* 23, 3–25.

6 Yamada, Y., Ito, K., Nakamura, K., Sawada, Y., Tatsuji, I. **1993**, *Biol. Pharm. Bull.* 16, 1251–1259.

7 Meir, J. **1982**, *Am. Heart J.* 104, 364–373.

8 Hinderling, P.H., Schmidlin, O., Seydel, J.K. **1984**, *J. Bipharm. Pharmacokinet.* 2, 263–286.

9 Taylor, D.C, Pownall, R., Burke, W. **1984**, *J. Pharm. Pharmacol.* 37, 280–283.

10 Arendt, R.M., Greenblatt, D.J., deJong, R.H., Bonin, J.D., Abernethy, D.R. **1984**, *Cardiology* 71, 307–314.

11 Johnsson, G., Regardh, C.-G. **1976**, *Clin. Pharmacokin.* 1, 233–263.

12 Ochs, H.R., Greenblatt, D.J., Arendt, R.M., Schafer-Korting, M., Mutschler, E. **1985**, *Arzneim.-Forsch./Drug Res.* 35, 1580–1582.

13 Upthagrove, A.L., Nelson, W.L. **2001**, *Drug Metab. Dispos.* 29, 1389–1395.

14 Beresford, A.P., Macrae, P.V., Stopher, D.A. **1988**, *Xenobiotica* 18, 169–182.

15 Bailey, D.G., Bend, J.R., Arnold, J.M., Tran, L.T., Spence, J.D. **1996**, *Clin. Pharmacol. Ther.*, 60, 25–33.

16 Brammer, K.W., Tarbit, M.H. **1988**, in *Recent trends in the discovery, development and evaluation of anti-fungal agents*, Fromtling, R.A. (ed.) JR Prous, Barcelona.

6
Renal Clearance

6.1
Kidney Anatomy and Function

The kidney can be subdivided in terms of anatomy and function into a series of units termed nephrons. The nephron consists of the glomerulus, proximal tubule, loop of Henle, distal tubule and the collecting tubule. Filtration by the glomerulus of plasma water is the first step in urine formation. A large volume of blood, approximately 1 L min^{-1} (or 25% of the entire cardiac output at rest) flows through the kidneys. Thus in four to five minutes a volume of blood equal to the total blood volume passes through the renal circulation, of this volume approximately 10% is filtered at the glomerulus. Small molecules are also filtered at this site. The concentration of drug is identical to that present unbound in plasma ($C_{p(f)}$). The rate at which plasma water is filtered (125 mL min^{-1}) is termed the glomerular filtration rate (GFR). In addition to the passive filtration, active secretion may also occur. Various transport proteins are present in the proximal tubule which are selective for acidic and basic compounds (ionised at physiological pH) [1]. For acidic compounds (organic anions), the transporter is located at the contraluminal cell membrane and uptake is a tertiary, active transport process. Physicochemical properties that determine affinity for this transporter are lipophilicity, ionic charge strength (decreasing the pK_a increases the affinity for the transporter) and electron attracting functions in the compound structure. The lipophilic region must have a minimal length of 4 Å and can be up to 10 Å. In addition hydrogen-bond formation increases the affinity for the transporter, and there is a direct relationship between the number of H-bond acceptors and affinity. A transport system for basic compounds (organic cations) is situated at the contraluminal membrane. Lipophilicity and ionic charge strength (increasing the pK_a increases affinity for the transporter) govern affinity. The transporter can also transport unionised compounds that have hydrogen-bonding functionality. At the luminal membrane an electroneutral H$^+$ organic cation transporter is also present. Compounds such as verapamil have similar affinity for this transporter compared to the contraluminal system, whilst cimetidine has higher affinity for it. Unlike glomerular filtration, all the blood passing through the kidney has access to the transporter so clearance rates can be much higher than GFR.

Pharmacokinetics and Metabolism in Drug Design.
Dennis A. Smith, Han van de Waterbeemd, Don K. Walker (Eds.)
Copyright © 2006 WILEY-VCH Verlag GmbH & Co. KGaA, Weinheim
ISBN: 3-527-31368-0

6.2
Lipophilicity and Reabsorption by the Kidney

Reabsorption, as highlighted previously, is the most important factor controlling the renal handling of drugs. The degree of reabsorption depends on the physico-chemical properties of the drug, principally its degree of ionisation and intrinsic lipophilicity (log D). The membranes of the cells that form the tubule are lipoidal (as expected) and do not represent a barrier to lipophilic molecules. Reabsorption occurs all along the nephron. Reabsorption re-establishes the equilibrium between the unbound drug in the urine (largely the case) and the unbound drug in plasma. As the kidney reabsorbs water so the drug is concentrated and hence if lipophilic, reabsorbed by passive diffusion. The majority (80–90%) of filtered water is reabsorbed in the proximal tubule. Most of the remainder is reabsorbed in the distal tubule and collecting ducts. From initial filtration the urine is concentrated approximately 100-fold. We can thus expect for neutral compounds renal clearance (unbound values) to range between GFR, for compounds that are not reabsorbed, and a value some 100-fold below this for compounds that are completely reabsorbed to an equilibrium with free drug in plasma. Figure 6.1 illustrates this relationship between lipophilicity and renal clearance for a series of neutral compounds.

Clearly, the ability to cross membranes, as represented by octanol partitioning correlates with the extent of reabsorption, with reabsorption only occurring at log $D_{7.4}$ values above zero.

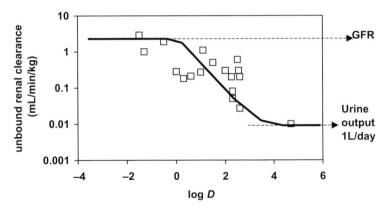

Fig. 6.1 Relationship between lipophilicity and unbound renal clearance (highlighting GFR and urine output) for a series of neutral drugs in man.

6.3
Effect of Charge on Renal Clearance

Similar patterns occur for acidic and basic drugs, however, tubular pH is often more acidic (pH 6.5) than plasma. Because of this, acidic drugs are reabsorbed more extensively and basic drugs less extensively than their log $D_{7.4}$ would suggest. Moreover, much greater rates of excretion/clearance can occur for these charged moieties due to the tubular active transport proteins. The effects of tubular secretion are particularly apparent as lipophilicity increases (as indicated by the structural features required by the transport systems described above), but before substantial tubular reabsorption occurs. With the shift in tubular pH, the value of zero as a threshold for reabsorption for neutral drugs (see Fig. 6.1) correlates to a value of –1 for acid drugs and +1 for basic drugs. These effects are illustrated in Fig. 6.2.

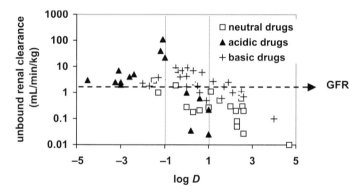

Fig. 6.2 Relationship between lipophilicity, GFR and unbound renal clearance for neutral , acidic and basic drugs in man.

Figure 6.2 highlights the role of lipophilicity in the active transport of drugs. Peak values for renal clearance for these compounds occur at log $D_{7.4}$ values between –2 and 0. These values span the region where the compounds have sufficient lipophilicity to interact with the transport proteins but are not substantially reabsorbed.

6.4
Plasma Protein Binding and Renal Clearance

As only the unbound drug is available for renal clearance by filtration at the glomerulus, drugs with high plasma protein binding will only appear slowly in the filtrate. Hence, considerations of the renal clearance process based on total drug concentrations either in plasma or urine may be misleading.

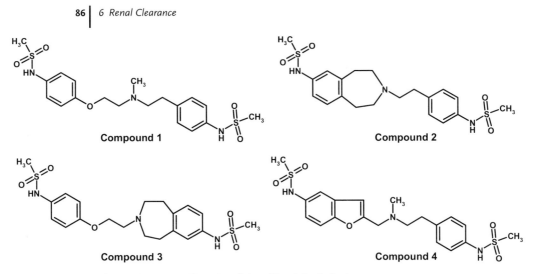

Fig. 6.3 Structures of a series of class III anti-dysrhythmic agents.

For example, a series of class III anti-dysrhythmic agents (Fig. 6.3) exhibited decreasing renal clearance in the dog with increasing lipophilicity over a log $D_{7.4}$ range 0.7 to 2.1 [2].

However, the major contributing factor to the decreased renal clearance of total drug was increasing plasma protein binding with increasing lipophilicity. When the extent of plasma protein binding was taken into account, the unbound renal clearance for the three least lipophilic compounds was virtually identical at around 6 mL per min per kg as shown in Fig. 6.4.

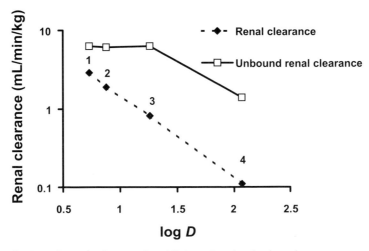

Fig. 6.4 Relationship between lipophilicity and total and unbound renal clearance in the dog for a series of class III anti-dysrhythmic agents (compounds 1 to 4 in Fig. 6.3).

The value for unbound renal clearance of 6 mL per min per kg is in excess of *GFR* in the dog (~4 mL per min per kg) indicating a degree of tubular secretion in the renal clearance of these basic molecules (pK_a values of 7.8–8.2). The unbound renal clearance of compound 4 is about 1.5 mL per min per kg and indicates substantial tubular reabsorption of this the most lipophilic member of the series. This compound is also substantially less basic than the others (pK_a of 7.3) and as such may be subject to reduced tubular secretion.

6.5
Balancing Renal Clearance and Absorption

As a clearance route the renal route has attractive features for the design of drugs. For instance clearance rates, certainly for neutral compounds, are low. Moreover, the clearance process by filtration is not saturable and tubular secretion is only saturated at high doses with acidic and basic compounds. In a similar vein, drug interactions also only occur at high doses for acidic and basic compounds and will not occur for neutral compounds. Renal function is also easily measured in patients (creatinine clearance) so variation in the process due to age or disease can be readily adjusted for by modification of the dosage regimen. On the negative side, low lipophilicity is usually necessary for the renal route to predominate over the metabolic route (see Chapter 5, Fig. 5.7). This requirement means that oral absorption of such compounds is likely to be via the paracellular pathway (see Chapter 3). This trend is highlighted in Table 6.1. In this table, the extent of renal clearance of compounds, previously exemplified in Chapter 3, as those absorbed by the paracellular route, is listed. Hence the positive aspects of clearance predominantly by the renal route have to be carefully balanced against the negative aspects of absorption by the paracellular pathway.

Tab. 6.1 Correlation between para-cellular absorption and renal clearance.

Compound	Log $D_{7.4}$	% Renally cleared
Atenolol	−1.5	85
Practolol	−1.3	95
Sotalol	−1.7	80
Xamoterol	−1.0	60
Nadolol	−2.1	65
Sumatriptan	−0.8	25
Pirenzipine	−0.6	40
Famotidine	−0.6	88
Ranitidine	−0.3	70
Amosulalol	−0.8	34

6.6
Renal Clearance and Drug Design

Small molecules with relatively simple structures (molecular weights below 350) can successfully combine paracellular absorption and renal clearance. Table 6.1 lists examples of this. Noticeably the compounds are all peripherally acting G-protein coupled receptor antagonists. When a compound has to cross membrane barriers to access an intracellular target (see Chapter 2, Section 2.10) or cross the blood-brain barrier, then these physicochemical properties are generally unsuitable. It is possible to design molecules of high metabolic stability that *defy* the general trends shown in Fig. 5.7.

Fluconazole (Fig. 6.5) is an example where knowledge of the relationship between physicochemical properties and drug disposition has allowed optimisation of the drug'performance [3]. The project goal was a superior compound to ketoconazole, the first orally active azole anti-fungal drug. Ketoconazole (Fig. 6.5) is cleared primarily by hepatic metabolism and shows irregular bioavailability, due partly to this, and also its poor aqueous solubility and consequent erratic dissolution. Ketoconazole is a neutral molecule with a log $D_{7.4}$ value greater than 4.0. The high lipophilicity leads to its dependence upon metabolic clearance and its low solubility.

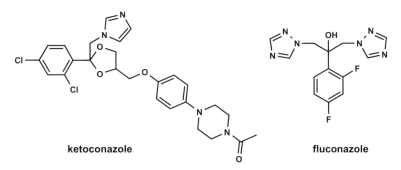

Fig. 6.5 Structures of the anti-fungal agents, ketoconazole and fluconazole.

Synthesis was directed towards metabolic stability and this was found in the bis-triazole series of compounds. Metabolic stability is achieved by the relative resistance of the triazole moiety to oxidative attack, the presence of halogen functions on the phenyl grouping, another site of possible oxidative attack and steric hindrance of the hydroxy function, a site for possible conjugation.

Due to the metabolic stability, low molecular weight and absence of ionisation at physiological pH, fluconazole has to rely on renal clearance as its major clearance mechanism. The compound has a log P or $D_{7.4}$ value of 0.5, which means following filtration at the glomerulus a substantial proportion (80%) of the compound in the filtrate will undergo tubular reabsorption. The resultant low rate of renal clearance gives fluconazole a 30 hour half-life in man and is consequently suitable for once a day administration.

References

1 Ullrich, K.J. **1994**, *Biochim. Biophys. Acta* 1197, 45–62.

2 Walker, D.K., Beaumont, K.C., Stopher, D.A., Smith, D.A. **1996**, *Xenobiotica* 26, 1101–1111.

3 Smith, D.A., Jones, B.C., Walker, D.K. **1996**, *Med. Res. Rev.* 16, 243–266.

7
Metabolic (Hepatic) Clearance

7.1
Function of Metabolism (Biotransformation)

Drug metabolism is traditionally divided into phase I and phase II processes. This classical division into primarily oxidative and conjugative processes, whilst useful, is not definitive. The division is based on the observation that a compound will first undergo oxidative attack (e.g. benzene to phenol), and then the newly introduced hydroxyl function will undergo glucuronidation (phenol to phenyl glucuronic acid). A listing of typical enzymes assigned to phase I and phase II is provided in Table 7.1.

Tab. 7.1 Division of enzymes into phase I and phase II. Phase I enzymes are normally oxidative and phase II conjugative.

Cytochrome P450 mono-oxygenase	Phase I
Azo and nitro group reductase	
Aldehyde dehydrogenase	
Alcohol dehydrogenase	
Epoxide hydrolase	
Monoamine oxidase	
Flavin monoamine oxidase	
Non-specific esterases	
Non-specific N-and O-methyl transferases	Phase II
D-glucuronic acid transferase	
Catechol-O-methyl transferase	
Glutathione transferase	
Sulphate transferase	

As was shown previously for SM-10888 compounds do not necessarily have to undergo phase I metabolism prior to phase II processes. Either or both (as with SM-10888) can be involved in the primary clearance of a drug. However, in gen-

Pharmacokinetics and Metabolism in Drug Design.
Dennis A. Smith, Han van de Waterbeemd, Don K. Walker (Eds.)
Copyright © 2006 WILEY-VCH Verlag GmbH & Co. KGaA, Weinheim
ISBN: 3-527-31368-0

eral, phase I enzymes are normally of greater import with the cytochrome P450 system occupying a pivotal role in drug clearance. Cytochrome P450 is a heme containing superfamily of enzymes. The superfamily consists of isoenzymes that are highly selective for endogenous substrates and isoenzymes that are less selective and metabolise exogenous substrates including drugs.

7.2
Cytochrome P450

The cytochrome P450 system can carry out a variety of oxidation reactions as listed below in Table 7.2.

Tab. 7.2 Reactions performed by the cytochrome P450 system.

Reaction	Product	Typical example
Aromatic hydroxylation	Phenyl to phenol	Phenytoin
Aliphatic hydroxylation	Methyl to carbinol	Ibuprofen
N-dealkylation	3° to 2° Amine	Lidocaine
O-dealkylation	Ether to alcohol	Naproxen
S-dealkylation	Thioether to thiol	6-Methylthiopurine
N-oxidation	Pyridine to pyridine N-oxide	Voriconazole
S-oxidation	Sulphoxide to sulphone	Omeprazole
Alcohol oxidation	Alcohol to carboxylic acid	Losartan

The overall scheme for these reactions is the insertion of a single oxygen atom into the drug molecule. Current views indicate that the chemistry of cytochrome P450 is radical by nature.

The mechanism of cytochrome P450 catalysis is probably constant across the system. It is determined by the ability of a high valent formal $(FeO)^{3+}$ species to carry out one-electron oxidations through the abstraction of hydrogen atoms or electrons. The resultant substrate radical can then recombine with the newly created hydroxyl radical (oxygen rebound) to form the oxidised metabolite. Where a heteroatom is the (rich) source of the electron more than one product is possible. There can be direct recombination to yield the heteroatom oxide or radical relocalisation within the substrate to an a-carbon, and oxidation of this function to form the unstable carbinol and ultimately heteroatom dealkylation. A possible reaction sequence is illustrated as Fig. 7.1.

Much of the investigations into the enzymology of cytochrome P450 over the previous 20 years has focused on the pathway that generates this reactant species as illustrated in Fig. 7.2, particularly the donation of electrons and protons to yield the $(FeO)^{3+}$-substrate complex that is the oxidising species. As part of the cycle

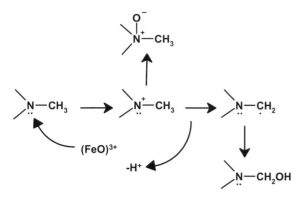

Fig. 7.1 Heteroatom oxidation of drugs by cytochrome P450 leading to heteroatom oxides or dealkylation products.

substrate binds to the enzyme as an initial step before the addition of electrons and molecular oxygen. The final stage of the cycle is the actual attack of the $(FeO)^{3+}$ species on the substrate.

The critical points of the cycle involving substrate–enzyme interactions are illustrated if Fig. 7.2 and explored below:

1. The initial binding of the substrate to the CYP, which causes a change in the spin state of the heme iron eventually resulting in the formation of the $(FeO)^{3+}$-substrate complex. This is obviously a key substrate–protein interaction and depends on the actual 3D structure of the substrate and the topography of the active site. However, it cannot be assumed that this initial binding is the same as the final confirmation that the protein and substrate adopt during actual substrate attack.

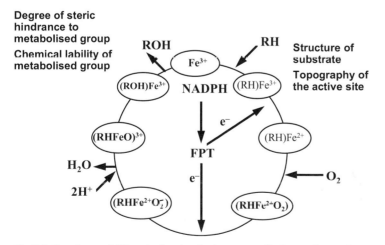

Fig. 7.2 Cytochrome P450 cycle showing the key stages of substrate interaction.

2. The final stages of the cycle are when the geometry and chemical reactivity of this complex determine the structure of the metabolite produced.

Analysis of the literature indicates that three major forms of CYPs are involved in the metabolism of pharmaceuticals in man: CYP2D6, CYP2C9 and CYP3A4 (CYP1A2, CYP2C19 and CYP2E1 are also involved, but this involvement is much less extensive). The catalytic selectivity of the major CYPs has been reviewed [1]. Although there is overlap between substrates for the CYPs, broad substrate–structure classifications can be made. These are outlined below before a more detailed description is given for three of the major forms:

- CYP1A2: Neutral or basic lipophilic planar molecules with at least one putative H-bond donating site. Principle substrate is theophylline.
- CYP2D6: Arylalkylamines (basic) with site of oxidation a discrete distance from a protonated nitrogen. Substrates are lipophilic, particularly when measured or calculated for the neutral form. Principle substrates are β-adrenoceptor blockers, class I anti-arrhythmics and tricyclic anti-depressants. Often hydroxylation occurs in an aromatic ring or an accompanying short alkyl side chain.
- CYP2C9: Neutral or acidic molecules with site of oxidation a discrete distance from H-bond donor or possibly anionic heteroatom. Molecules tend to be amphipathic with a region of lipophilicity at the site of hydroxylation and an area of hydrophobicity around the H-bond forming region. Principal substrates are non-steroidal anti-inflammatory agents. Oxidation often occurs in an aromatic ring or an accompanying short alkyl side chain.
- CYP3A4: Lipophilic, neutral, or basic molecules with site of oxidation often nitrogen (N-dealkylation) or allylic positions. Wide range of substrates covering all fields of pharmaceuticals.
- CYP2E1: Small (molecular weight of 200 Da or less) normally lipophilic linear and cyclic molecules. Principle pharmaceutical compounds are volatile anaesthetics.

7.2.1
Catalytic Selectivity of CYP2D6

Substrates for CYP2D6 include tricyclic anti-depressants, β-blockers, class I anti-arrhythmics. In brief, the structural similarities of many of the substrates and inhibitors in terms of position of hydroxylation overall structure (arylalkylamine) and physicochemistry (ionised nitrogen at physiological pH) have allowed template models such as that illustrated as Fig. 7.3 to be constructed.

All the template models produced have the same common features of a basic nitrogen atom at a distance of 5–7 Å from the site of metabolism, which is in gen-

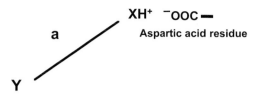

a

XH+ ⁻OOC —

Aspartic acid residue

Y

Fig. 7.3 Template model for CYP2D6 with Y the site of oxidation, a is the distance from Y to a heteroatom which is positively charged (normally 5–7 Å).

eral on or near a planar aromatic system. It is currently believed that glutamic acid residue 216 and aspartic acid residue 301 provide the carboxylate residues which binds the basic nitrogen of the substrates [2].

With CYP2D6 therefore the catalytic selectivity relies heavily on a substrate–protein interaction. The relative strength of the proposed ion pair between the basic nitrogen and the active site aspartic acid means that the affinity for substrates will be high. This is borne out by the enzyme having lower K_m and K_i (binding constant) values than other CYPs. Thus CYP2D6 is often a major enzyme in drug oxidation despite its low abundance in the human liver. This statement is particularly true for low concentrations or doses of drugs, the low K_m values rendering the enzyme easily saturable (see Section 2.12). An example of this is the antiarrhythmic compound propafenone (Fig. 7.4) [3], which is converted to 5-hydroxy propafenone by CYP2D6.

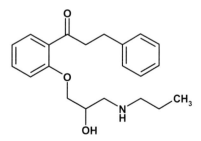

Fig. 7.4 Structure of propafenone.

The dependence on CYP2D6 metabolism and the relatively high clinical dose (see Fig. 7.5) mean that the metabolism is readily saturable over a narrow clinical dose range, so that small increases in dose can lead to disproportionate increases in plasma concentration, and a resultant steep dose response curve.

CYP2D6 is also problematic in drug therapy since the enzyme is absent in about 7% of Caucasians due to genetic polymorphism. In these 7% (poor metabolisers) clearance of CYP2D6 substrates such as propafenone (Fig. 7.4) [4] are markedly lower and can lead to side effects in these subsets of the population. This correlation of enhanced side effects in poor metabolisers (lacking CYP2D6)

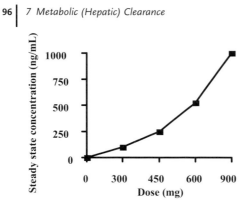

Fig. 7.5 Relationship between plasma concentration and dose for propafenone, a CYP2D6 substrate.

compared to extensive metabolisers (active CYP2D6) has been made for propafenone. The example of betaxolol shows how knowledge of the properties that bestow pharmacological activity can be combined with metabolism concepts to produce a molecule with improved performance [5].

Cardioselectivity for β-adrenoceptor agents can be conferred by substitution in the para-position of the phenoxypropanolamine skeleton. The para-position or methoxy ethyl substituents (e.g. metoprolol) in this position are the major sites of metabolism for these compounds. This reaction is catalysed by CYP2D6, and the efficiency of the enzyme means that metoprolol shows high clearance and resultant low bioavailability and short half-life. Manoury and colleagues [5] designed the series of compounds leading to betaxolol on the hypothesis that bulky stable substituents in the para-position (Fig. 7.6) would be resistant to metabolism and also cardioselective.

Beside the actual steric bulk of the substituent, cyclopropyl is much more stable to hydrogen abstraction than other alkyl functions and represents an ideal terminal group. These changes make betaxolol a compound with much improved pharmacokinetics compared to its lipophilic analogues.

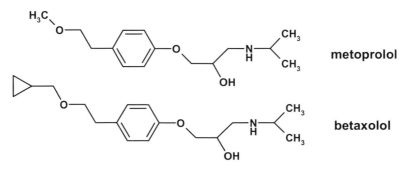

Fig. 7.6 Structures of metoprolol and betaxolol, an analogue designed to be more metabolically stable.

7.2.2
Catalytic Selectivity of CYP2C9

Substrates for CYP2C9 include many non-steroidal anti-inflammatories, plus a reasonably diverse set of compounds including phenytoin, (S)-warfarin and tolbutamide. All the substrates with routes of metabolism attributable to CYP2C9 have hydrogen bond donating groups a discrete distance from a lipophilic region, which is the site of hydroxylation. The hydrogen bond donating groups and sites of metabolism on each of the substrates have been overlayed with those of phenytoin to produce a putative template of the active site of CYP2C9 (Fig. 7.7).

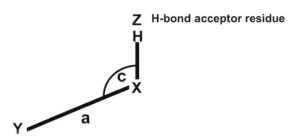

Fig. 7.7 Template model of CYP2C9, Y is the site of oxidation, *a* is the distance from Y to a heteroatom, which can act as an H-bond donor, and *c* defines the angle of the H-bond.

The mean dimensions ($\pm$ SD) for the eight compounds (a = 6.7 $\pm$ 0.8 Å, c = 133 $\pm$ 20°) illustrates the degree of overlap achieved. Like CYP2D6 the catalytic selectivity of CYP2C9 is dominated by substrate–protein interactions.

Tolbutamide (Fig. 7.8) is metabolised in the benzylic methyl group by CYP2C9 as the major clearance mechanism. Chlorpropamide is a related compound incorporating a chlorine function in this position. The resultant metabolic stability gives chlorpropamide a lower clearance and a longer half-life (approximately 35 hours compared to 5 hours) than tolbutamide, resulting in a substantial increase in duration of action [6].

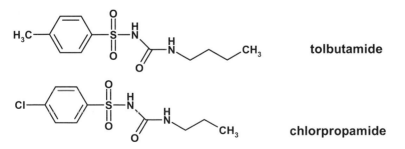

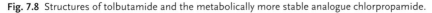

Fig. 7.8 Structures of tolbutamide and the metabolically more stable analogue chlorpropamide.

The mechanism of CYPs is radical rather than electrophilic and actual substitution pattern is important: the role of chlorine is one of blocking rather than deactivation. Many non-steroidal anti-inflammatory drugs are substrates for the CYP2C9 enzyme and analogous structures show how metabolic stability to *p*-hydroxylation is achieved with only small changes in substitution.

Diclofenac, with ortho-substitution in the aromatic ring (Fig. 7.9) is metabolised principally to 4-hydroxydiclofenac by CYP2C9. In man, the drug has a short half-life of approximately one hour due to the relatively high metabolic (oxidative) clearance. In contrast, the analogous compound, fenclofenac, is considerably more metabolically stable, due to the *p*-halogen substitution pattern, and exhibits a half-life of over 20 hours [7].

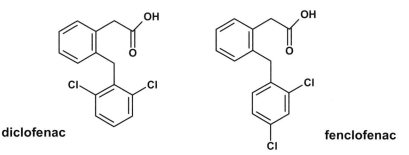

diclofenac   **fenclofenac**

Fig. 7.9 Structures of diclofenac and fenclofenac, fenclofenac is much more resistant to aromatic hydroxylation.

7.2.3
Catalytic Selectivity of CYP3A4

CYP3A4 metabolises lipophilic drugs in positions largely determined by their chemical lability, i.e. the ease of hydrogen or electron abstraction. CYP3A4 SAR is dominated therefore by substrate–reactant interactions. Binding of substrates seems to be essentially due to lipophilic forces and results in the expulsion of water from the active site. Such an expulsion of water provides the driving force for the spin state change and hence the formation of the $(FeO)^{3+}$ unit. However, the lipophilic forces holding the substrate in the active site are relatively weak ($\sim$1 Kcal mole^{-1}) and would allow motion of the substrate in the active site. Hence, since the substrate is able to adopt more than one orientation in the active site, the eventual product of the reaction is a product of the interaction between one of these orientations and the $(FeO)^{3+}$ unit, a substrate–reactant interaction. This lack of apparent substrate–structure similarity (apart from chemical reactivity) indicates a large active site that allows substrate molecules considerable mobility. The selectivity of CYP3A4 to its substrates may also be directed by the conformations they adopt within a lipophilic environment such as we are suggesting the access channel and active site of CYP3A4 to be. We have previously illustrated this point with cyclosporine A. In an aprotic (lipophilic solvent) cyclosporine A adopts a conformation which allows the major allylic site of CYP3A4 metabolism to extend out away from the bulk of the molecule. This is a different conformation from the one adopted in aqueous solution where the lipophilic site of metabolism are internalised, shielded from the solvent. As a general rule this *spreading out* of apparently sterically hindered molecules as judged by x-ray or aqueous solution structure may help to understand further the selectivity of CYP3A4. The principal of extension of lipophilic functions normally hidden from solvent is further supported by study of the soluble bacterial P450BM-3. In this case, the substrates are fatty acids, which in aqueous solution adopt a *globular* conformation. However, upon entering the lipophilic access channel of the fatty acid, it opens out in an extended conformation with the lipophilic head group directed at the heme and the polar acid function directed at the solvent.

The enzyme is the principal participant in *N*-demethylation reactions where the substrate is a tertiary amine. The list of substrates includes erythromycin, ethylmorphine, lidocaine, diltiazem, tamoxifen, toremifene, verapamil, cocaine, amiodarone, alfentanil and terfenadine. Allylic and benzylic position carbons, such as

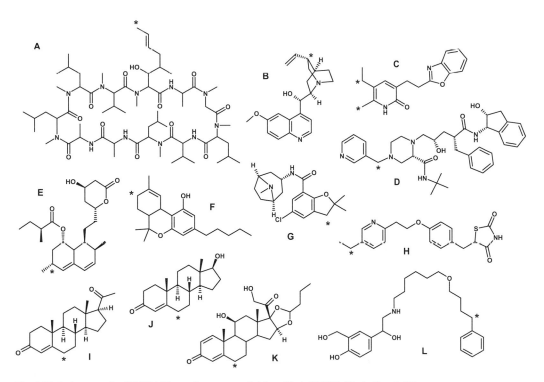

Fig. 7.10 Substrates for CYP3A4 illustrating the diversity of structure and the *selectivity* for metabolism at allylic and benzylic positions (major sites of metabolism indicated by asterisks). Substrates are cyclosporine A (A), quinidine (B), L-696229 (C), indinavir (D), lovastatin (E), Δ-THC (F), zatosetron (G), pioglitazone (H), progesterone (I), testosterone (J), budesonide (K) and salmeterol (L).

those present in quinidine, steroids and cyclosporine A, are also particularly prone to oxidation by CYP3A4. A range of substrates is illustrated in Fig. 7.10.

Both these routes reflect the ease of hydrogen or electron abstraction from these functions. As with conventional radical chemistry, reactivity needs to be combined with probability. Thus, in molecules such as terfenadine the tertiary butyl group will be liable to oxidation due to its *maximum number* of equivalent primary carbons. Thus, although not a specially labile function, the site of metabolism becomes dominated by statistical probability. Terfenadine, as expected, also undergoes N-dealkylation by CYP3A4 illustrating the ability of the enzyme to produce multiple products (as for cyclosporine A, midazolam, etc.) and underlining the *flexibility* of CYP3A4 substrate binding.

Recently the crystal structure of CYP3A4 has been obtained and confirmed many of the speculations [8]. The active site has a probe-accessible volume of $520 \, \text{Å}^3$. CYP3A4 is unique amongst P450 structurally characterised to date in having seven phenylalanine residues forming a *Phe-cluster*, which lie above the active site, with the aromatic side chains stacking against each other to form a hydrophobic core. The Phe-cluster results in a closed conformation of the active site. The heme of CYP3A4 has greater accessibility to the active site than comparable P450s, such as CYP2C9 (Fig. 7.11).

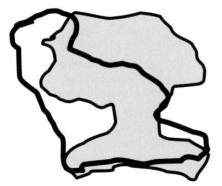

Fig. 7.11 Schematic showing the active site dimensions of CYP3A4 and CYP2C9 (grey shading). The heme is at the bottom of the active site and much more accessible in CYP3A4 than CYP2C9 despite their overall similar volumes.

This greater accessibility could allow two substrate molecules to have access to the reactive oxygen, explaining the observation that CYP3A4 is able to bind and simultaneously metabolise multiple substrates molecules. Moreover, the relative ease of access also explains how compounds can be metabolised at multiple sites by the enzyme with little apparent steric constraints. The crystal structure indicates that the binding of molecules will be primarily hydrophobic. Binding of a substrate or inhibitor involves the complete removal of the groups, at the binding interface, from water. The loss of solvent is a major contributor to the binding free energy. Lipophilic groups have a positive solvation free energy, this together with favourable direct van der Waals interactions, make lipophilic interactions a key force in binding. In contrast the desolvation of polar groups is unfavourable, although hydrogen bonds, etc., between the substrate and enzyme, are favourable. The contribution of polar contacts to the binding free energy is likely to be variable due to the balance of desolvation and actual binding. Figure 7.12 illustrates the relationship between K_m values of CYP3A4 substrates as a measure of affinity for the enzyme and lipophilicity and indicates the good correlation.

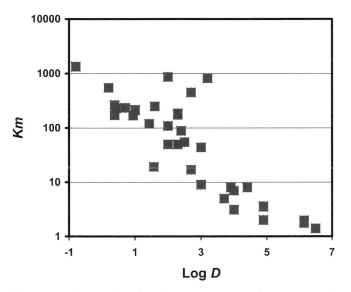

Fig. 7.12 Correlation of K_m values for various CYP3A4 substrates corrected for microsomal binding and lipophilicity (log $D_{7.4}$).

Overcoming metabolism by CYP3A4 is difficult due to the extreme range of substrates and the tolerance of the enzyme to structure. Two strategies are available: removal of functionality and reduction of lipophilicity.

Allylic and benzylic positions are points of metabolic vulnerability. SCH48461 was a potent cholesterol absorption inhibitor [9]. Metabolic attack was at a number of positions including benzylic hydroxylation. Dugar and co-workers substituted oxygen for the C-3'-carbon to remove this site of metabolism. This step however, produces an electron-rich phenoxy moiety in comparison to the original phenyl group and possibly made this function more amenable to aromatic hydroxylation. Blocking of the aromatic oxidation with fluorine introduced in the para-position was required to produce the eventual more stable substitution. These steps are shown in Fig. 7.13.

The lability of benzylic positions to cytochrome P450 metabolism has been exploited to decrease the unacceptably low clearance and resultant long half-life of compounds. For example celecoxib, a selective cyclooxygenase inhibitor, has a

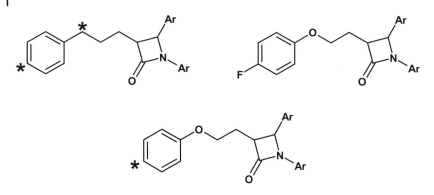

Fig. 7.13 Synthetic strategies to overcome benzylic hydroxylation in a series of cholesterol absorption inhibitors. Positions of metabolism are marked with an asterisk.

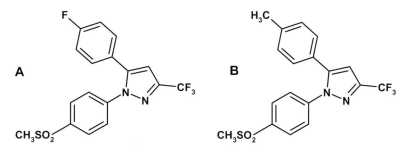

Fig. 7.14 Structures of early long half-life COX2 inhibitor (A) and the candidate celecoxib (B), a compound with a moderate half-life.

half-life of 3.5 hours in rats. Early structural leads, represented by compounds in which celecoxib's benzylic methyl was a halogen substituent (Fig. 7.14), had half-life values (in male rats) up to 220 hours [10].

Diltiazem (Fig. 7.15), a calcium channel blocker, is a drug that is extensively metabolised by at least five distinct pathways including *N*-demethylation, deacetylation, *O*-demethylation, ring hydroxylation and acid formation. The enzyme responsible for at least the major route (*N*-demethylation), has been shown to be CYP3A4. Although widely used in therapy, the compound has a relatively short duration of action. In the search for superior compounds, Floyd and colleagues [11] substituted the benzazepinone ring structure for the benzothiazepinone of diltiazem. Metabolism studies on this class of compound showed that the principal routes of metabolism were similar to that for diltiazem with *N*-demethylation, conversion to an aldehyde (precursor of an acid), deacetylation and *O*-demethylation all occurring. It was also noted that the *N*-desmethyl derivative was equipotent to the parent but much more metabolically stable. This can be rationalised as the decreased substitution on the nitrogen (2° versus 3°) stabilising the nitrogen

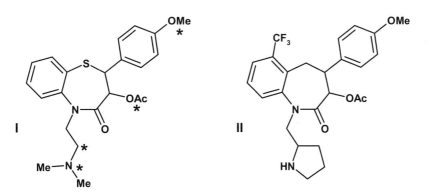

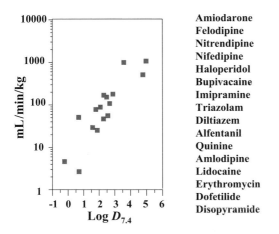

Fig. 7.15 Structures of diltiazem and a benzazepinone analogue resistant to metabolism.

to electron abstraction (decreased radical stability). This stabilisation is particularly important, since the electron abstraction is the first step to both the N-desmethyl and aldehyde products (a total of 84% of the total metabolism). The evidence of stability of secondary amines was capitalised on by synthesis of N-1 pyrrolidinyl derivatives, which were designed to achieve metabolic stability both by the decreased radical stability of secondary compounds to tertiary amines and steric hindrance afforded by β-substitution (Fig. 7.15). The success of this strategy indicates how even the vulnerable alkyl substituted nitrogen grouping can be stabilised to attack.

The predominant interaction of CYP3A4 is via hydrophobic forces and overall lowering of lipophilicity can reduce metabolic lability to the enzyme. Figure 7.16 shows the relationship between unbound intrinsic clearance in man and lipophili-

Amiodarone
Felodipine
Nitrendipine
Nifedipine
Haloperidol
Bupivacaine
Imipramine
Triazolam
Diltiazem
Alfentanil
Quinine
Amlodipine
Lidocaine
Erythromycin
Dofetilide
Disopyramide

Fig. 7.16 Unbound intrinsic clearance of CYP3A4 substrates and relationship with lipophilicity. The data has been calculated from various clinical studies with the drugs listed in order of decreasing lipophilicity.

city for a variety of CYP3A4 substrates. The substrates are cleared by a variety of metabolic routes including N-dealkylation, aromatisation, and aromatic and aliphatic hydroxylation. The trend for lower metabolic lability with lower lipophilicity holds regardless of structure and metabolic route.

7.3
Other Oxidative Metabolism Processes

Aldehyde oxidase is a member of a family of enzymes referred to as molybdenum cofactor-containing enzymes (which includes xanthine oxidase) due to the presence of the unique molybdopterin prosthetic group. It is an enzyme involved in the metabolism of drugs, and other xenobiotics that possess aldehyde and azaheterocyclic substituents, among others [12]. It is present in the liver, as well as some other tissues of humans and other mammalian species such as the rat, guinea pig, monkey, and rabbit. Aldehyde oxidase converts aldehydes to carboxylic acids and azaheterocyclic compounds to lactams using molecular oxygen as an electron acceptor. It can also catalyze reduction reactions of some drugs, with the drug that is reduced replacing oxygen as the electron acceptor. Although the number of drug substrates are few it assumes some importance due to the oxidation of certain heterocycles and the known species differences in activity.

An example of its role is shown in the metabolism of the hypnotic agent, zaleplon [13]. Aldehyde oxidase generates the major metabolite 5-oxozaleplon (Fig. 7.17) as well as the corresponding 5-oxo analogue of the N-dealkylated metabolite of zaleplon. It is notable that the metabolism is much faster in the cynomolgus monkey than the rat.

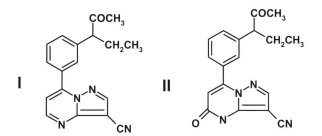

Fig. 7.17 Zaleplon a substrate for aldehyde oxidase (I) and the 5-oxo metabolite (II) formed by the enzyme.

Another drug example is the bioactivation of famciclovir to the active anti-viral agent penciclovir, which requires aldehyde oxidase-mediated metabolism [14]. Famciclovir is converted to the 6-oxo metabolite, which undergoes de-esterification to penciclovir; also, the de-esterified analogue of famciclovir, 6-deoxypenciclovir, is oxidized by aldehyde oxidase to the active compound. Although it is not frequently involved in initial pathways of metabolism of drugs, aldehyde oxidase may play a greater role in the intermediary metabolism of compounds, since aldehydes are frequent metabolic intermediates in the oxidative metabolism of alcohols to carboxylic acids [15].

SB-277011 is a dopamine D_3 receptor antagonist (Fig 7.18) with high oral bioavailability in the rat [16]. During the early development the previous high metabolic stability in rat, dog, cynomolgus monkey and human liver microsomes was not duplicated with whole liver homogenates from monkey and man. The 35-fold increase in intrinsic clearance was attributed to aldehyde oxidase. The rat has much lower rates of aldehyde oxidase metabolism. The predicted human bioavailability in contrast to the rat was very low, due to this species difference. The example illustrates the need to use an integrated metabolism system for screening at a fairly early stage to establish that the expected pathways are operational and unexpected pathways are not active (Section 10.6).

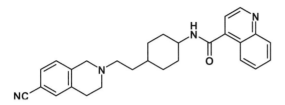

Fig. 7.18 SB-277011, a dopamine antagonist stable in liver microsomal metabolism systems, but a substrate for aldehyde oxidase.

The mammalian flavin mono-oxygenases (FMOs), like the P450s, although not as catalytically or structurally diverse as the P450 superfamily, are responsible for the conversion of lipophilic xenobiotics to more hydrophilic metabolites by the addition of oxygen through an NADPH-dependent pathway. Substrates for FMOs include several nitrogen and sulphur-containing compounds. Amines and sulfides are converted to N- and S-oxides. Five mammalian FMO isoforms have been identified and categorised through amino acid or cDNA sequencing as FMOs 1 to 5. Of these, FMO3 is the prominent form in the human liver. The mechanism of this flavoenzyme is unusual in that reduction of O_2 by nicotinamide adenine dinucleotide phosphate reduced (NADPH) occurs before the addition of the xenobiotic substrate (the loaded gun). Compounds bearing a soft nucleophilic heteroatom show substrate activity provided they contact the enzyme-bound 4a-hydroperoxy flavin. The amine nitrogen atom is not an especially soft nucleophile that is readily hydroxylated by peroxides or peracids. This grouping is a substrate, but how the enzyme converts an amine substrate to a form readily attacked by the hydroperoxy flavin is presently unknown. Structure–activity studies suggest that in addition to nucleophilicity, size and charge of potential substrates are important parameters limiting access to the enzyme-bound hydroxylating intermediate form of the enzyme. The mechanism of FMOs are similar and differences in the substrate specificities of these isoforms can be attributed almost entirely to differences in the dimensions of the access channel limiting access to the 4a hydroperoxy flavin.

Because of the nature of its substrates FMO metabolism normally occurs in tandem with cytochrome P450 metabolism and examples where it represents the major clearance pathway are relatively few. One example is itopride [17], which undergoes FMO catalysed N-oxidation as its major clearance route (Fig. 7.19). Although this route of metabolism has advantages from a drug interaction point of view (FMO unlikely to show significant drug interactions unlike P450, see Section 8.14), FMO is still subject to genetic polymorphisms and significant population differences in pharmacokinetic properties are likely to be observed in compounds metabolised by FMO3.

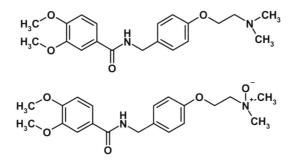

Fig. 7.19 Itopride (a substrate for FMO3) and its N-oxide metabolite. Itopride represents the relative minority of drugs cleared predominantly by FMO metabolism.

Monoamine oxidases (MAO-A and MAO-B) are well recognised in medicinal chemistry as proven drug targets. The enzymes can play a role in the endogenous metabolism of drugs. The enzymes are mitochondrial outer membrane-bound flavoproteins that catalyse the oxidative deamination of primary aliphatic and aromatic amines as well as some secondary and tertiary amines [18]. The reaction involves the binding of substrate to the enzyme before oxygen (contrast with FMO above). The reaction proceeds in two stages: reduction of the enzyme-bound FAD results in formation of the aldehyde product, followed by the second step of reoxidation of the enzyme-bound FAD by O_2 and the formation of hydrogen peroxide. For a primary amine, for instance, the reaction proceeds via an imine, which is hydrolysed to the final product:

$$R\underset{NH_2}{\overset{H_2}{C}} \xrightarrow{-2H} R\underset{NH}{\overset{H}{C}} \xrightarrow{+H_2O} R\underset{O}{\overset{H}{C}} + NH_3$$

At the α-position, with respect to the nitrogen atom, the pro-R-hydrogen is removed both by MAO-A and -B. At the β-position, MAO-A seems to recognise, as a substrate, only the R form, whereas MAO-B oxidizes both the R and S enantiomers. Compared with MAO-A substrates, a higher lipophilicity appears to characterise the typical MAO-B substrates. Of particular note with drug substrates are the triptans: sumatriptan, zolmitriptan and rizatriptan and the β-adrenoceptor agonists and antagonists such as propranolol, metoprolol, alprenolol, oxprenolol and timolol [19]. Most drugs do not have MAO catalysed metabolism as a primary clearance pathway (e.g. β-adrenoceptor agonists and antagonists), but for the cited triptans above, MAO is the primary metabolic clearance. This finding probably reflects the low lipophilicity of these triptans and their stability to oxidative enzymes such as P450. The log $D_{7.4}$ value of sumatriptan is around −1.7 and there is no evidence of P450 involvement [20]. MAO-A catalyses the metabolism of sumatriptan to an aldehyde product, which is converted to the final indole acetic acid (Fig. 7.20). Unusually for such a hydrophobic compound, the hepatic extraction by metabolism in human by MAO is such that the absorption of at least 57% is attenuated to a bioavailability of 14% [21]. The large effects on bioavailability can be attributed to a relatively low intrinsic clearance by MAO, but very low plasma protein binding (see Section 2.3) due to the low lipophilicity.

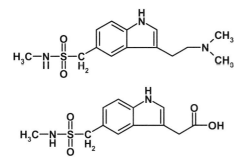

Fig. 7.20 Sumatriptan (a substrate for MAO-A) and its primary indole acetic acid metabolite.

7.4
Oxidative Metabolism and Drug Design

Besides the examples indicated above the design of orally active cholesterol absorption inhibitors combines both the concept of preventing metabolism and the serendipity of metabolites being more active than the parent drug [22]. On the basis of metabolite structure–activity relationships for SCH 48461 (Fig. 7.21), SCH 58335 was designed to combine activity enhancing oxidations and to remove or block sites of detrimental metabolic oxidations. The improvement in the pharmacodynamics of the compound is illustrated by the ED_{50} being reduced for the cholesterol hamster model from 2.2 to 0.04 mg per kg per day.

The discovery of the potassium channel opener cromakalim is another example of metabolism providing novel active molecules [23]. The programme was trying to seek agents that were anti-hypertensive without β-adrenoceptor blocking activity. This was due to the belief that β-adrenoceptor blockade was not solely responsible for the anti-hypertensive effects of β-adrenoceptor blockers. Early compounds were synthesised as cyclized derivatives of β-adrenoceptor blockers. The initial lead is illustrated in Fig. 7.22. The gem-dimethyl group and an electron-withdrawing group on the aromatic ring were essential. Cyclic amino groups were preferred to the original isopropylamine, leading to the pyrrolidine derivative. The eventual candidate cromakalim was produced by investigating the metabolites of the pyrrolidine derivative, an oxidation to amines to produce amides being a common metabolic step in cyclic amide systems.

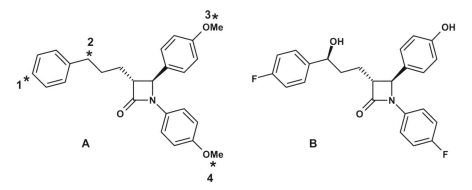

Fig. 7.21 Structures of cholesterol absorption inhibitors SCH 48461 (A) and SCH 58235 (B). Metabolism of SCH 48461 occurs by aromatic hydroxylation (1), benzylic hydroxylation (2), and O-demethylation (3,4) and is blocked in SCH 58235 at 1 and 4 or increases potency 2 and 3.

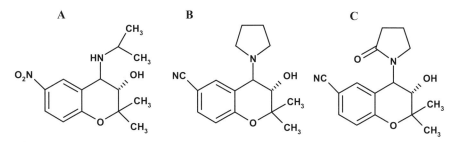

Fig. 7.22 Steps in the discovery of cromakalim: initial lead (A), more potent pyrrolidine analogue (B) and active metabolite (cromakalim, C).

7.5
Non-Specific Esterases

7.5.1
Function of Esterases

Non-specific esterases are distributed widely throughout the body. The activity of these enzymes varies markedly with different tissues. In mammals the highest levels are found in the liver and kidney. Numerous isoenzymes exist which have broad substrate overlap. A loose categorisation divides the two enzyme types likely to be involved in drug hydrolysis into arylesterases and aliesterases. Aliesterases have a wide substrate range, arylesterases require a phenolic ester. Since most of the important tissues contain a mixture, this division is not of great importance. Where esters are of great benefit to drug design is in the design of rapidly cleared molecules, either to an inactive or active form. The most rapid clearance is by blood metabolism. An important point in the screening of compounds designed for rapid metabolism is that the erythrocyte surface has high esterase content and whole blood is therefore the medium of choice. Moreover, rodent blood has very high esterase content, and may give a misleading view of stability if this species is used in isolation. It is highly likely that many of these enzymes are serine esterases and a suggested mechanism is proposed in Fig. 7.23.

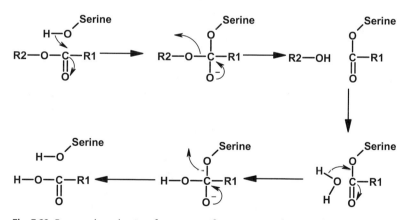

Fig. 7.23 Proposed mechanism for non-specific esterase catalysis involving a serine residue.

Ester functions present in molecules tend to be considered labile, although steric effects, etc., may be utilised to produce drugs without inherent chemical or metabolic problems due to ester lability. For instance, a series of antimuscarinic compounds which had selectivity for the M3 receptor (Fig. 7.24) were stabilised by the incorporation of a hydroxyethyl side chain or a cyclic ring system at position surrounding the ester function. Presumably, the proximity of these groups to the ester function (carbonyl) prevents close approach of the *attacking* nucleophile, in this case probably a serine hydroxyl.

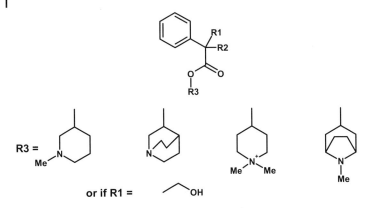

Fig. 7.24 Stabilisation of antimuscarinic compounds to esterase activity by steric effects. Stability was achieved when groupings corresponding to those illustrated were incorporated.

7.5.2
Ester Drugs as Intravenous and Topical Agents

The lability can be used as an advantage to create drugs that are designed for topical or intravenous infusion administration. For topical administration compounds can benefit from rapid systemic clearance to overcome possible side effects. Thus the compound is stable at its topical site of action (skin, eye, etc.) but rapidly degraded by the esterases present in blood, liver and kidneys to inactive metabolites. This approach renders the compound selective.

The aim of intravenous infusion is often to achieve a steady state plasma concentration as rapidly as possible, and as importantly, to have a drug whose concentrations decline as rapidly as possible once the infusion is stopped. This gives the clinician complete control and an ability to react quickly to patient needs. Figure 7.25 shows how existing drugs such as the anaesthetic/analgesic sulfentanil, the β-blocker propranolol and the ACE inhibitor captopril, have been used as the starting point for the design of short-acting infusion agents. A key to this design is the need for the acid metabolites produced from ester hydrolysis to be devoid of activity. In the case of remifentanil two sites of hydrolysis were incorporated to provide sufficient metabolic lability [24, 25].

Topical agents can also be produced by the *soft-drug* approach. Bodor [26] has produced methatropine and methscopolamine soft analogues. These are potent anti-cholinergics with a short duration of mydriatic action. Moreover, the compounds show no systemic side effects. They thus have a highly selective local action with a much decreased potential for systemic side effects. Again the design of these drugs depends on the knowledge that the acidic metabolites produced are inactive.

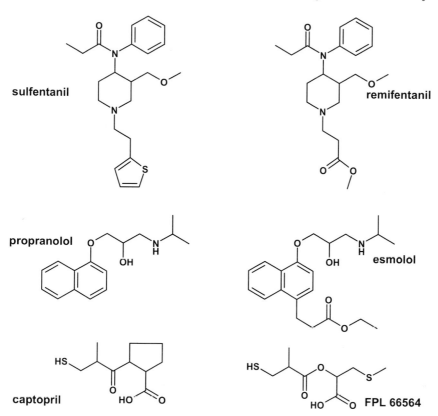

Fig. 7.25 Design of rapidly cleared ester analogues of sulfentanil, propranolol, and captopril. The compounds remifentanil, esmolol and FPL 66564 are all cleared to inactive metabolites.

7.6
Prodrugs to Aid Membrane Transfer

The esterification of a carboxylic acid function in a molecule has the immediate effect of a reduction in H-bonding potential and an increase in lipophilicity. Such parameters are important in the oral absorption of compounds as described before. Candoxatrilat (Fig. 7.26), an inhibitor of neutral endopeptidase (NEP), has poor oral bioavailability [27]. The compound has a log D of −2. The indanyl ester analogue candoxatril (Fig. 7.26) has an increased lipophilicity with a log D of 1.5, and a reduced H-bonding potential as reflected by its Raevsky score [27]. As such the compound is well within the properties expected for an oral agent. The pro-drug is well absorbed, rapidly hydrolysed but complete conversion is not achieved. The proportion of candoxatrilat liberated depends on competing clearance processes for candoxatril clearance, e.g. hepatic uptake/biliary clearance. For candoxatrilat the values of systemic availability after oral administration to mouse, rat, dog and man are 88, 53, 17 and 32%, and depend on the esterase activity (of which rodents are the highest) and the competing processes (of which man is probably the lowest).

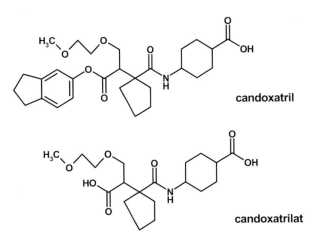

Fig. 7.26 Structures of candoxatril, the orally absorbed indanyl ester prodrug of candoxatrilat.

7.7
Enzymes Catalysing Drug Conjugation

7.7.1
Glucuronyl and Sulpho-Transferases

One of the most important phase II conjugation reactions is that catalysed by the glucuronyl-transferases. A number of functional groups have the potential to be glucuronidated as shown in Table 7.3, but phenol and carboxylic acid functions are of prime importance to the medicinal chemist.

Tab. 7.3 Reactions performed by the glucuronyl transferases.

Function	Typical example
Aliphatic hydroxyl	Tiaramide
Phenol	Morphine
Aromatic carboxyl	Furosemide
Aromatic tetrazole	Losartan
Aliphatic carboxyl	Benoxaprofen
Imidazole	Tioconazole
Aromatic amine	Dapsone
Tertiary amine	Chlorpromazine
Triazine	Lamotrigine

Glucuronidation involves the transfer of D-glucuronic acid from UDP-α-glucuronic acid to an acceptor compound. The family of enzymes that catalyse this reaction are the UDP-glucuronyl-transferases [28]. The reaction proceeds by nucleophilic S_N2 substitution of the C-1'-carbon of glucuronic acid, the product undergoing inversion of configuration. The mechanism is illustrated schematically in Fig.7.27.

Deprotonation

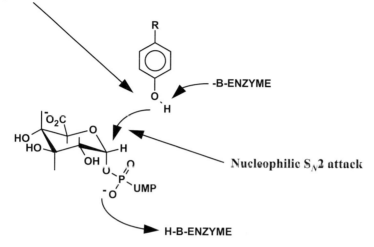

Fig. 7.27 Schematic showing mechanism of glucuronidation reactions.

Similar mechanisms apply to sulphate transferases, in which the donor is 3'-phosphoadenosine-5-phosphosulphate (PAPS). The accepting groups in the molecule are phenols, alcohols and hydroxylamines. The sulpho-transferases are relatively non-specific, however, phenol-sulpho-transferase is probably the most relevant to the medicinal chemist. The similarity in mechanism [29, 30] is shown by comparing the V_{max} values for glucuronyl-transferase and sulpho-transferase for a series of power substituted phenols. Figure 7.28 shows the log V_{max} for these series plotted against the Hammett sigma value.

The negative slope of both curves indicates the greater the nucleophilicity (electron donating ability) of the phenolate anion the faster the rate of the reaction. The initial deprotonation of the phenol is apparently not rate-limiting and must occur rapidly for those compounds with pK_a values high enough to require deprotonation. Recently x-ray crystal structure information [31, 32] has been obtained for various sulpho-transferases. The active site (Fig 7.29) comprises a hydrophobic pocket of phenylalanine residue. In the case of the catechol transferase SULT1A3 a glutamic acid residue provides an ion-pair interaction with the basic nitrogen of many of its natural substrates such as dopamine. A critical residue in the catalytic process is a lysine which stabilises the transition state and via a hydrogen-bond interaction with the bridge oxygen, between the 5'-phosphate group and the sul-

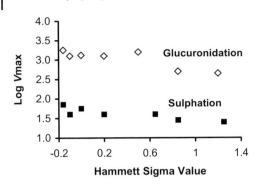

Fig. 7.28 Relationship between sigma value and enzyme rate for glucuronyl and sulpho-transferases indicating the role of nucleophilicity.

phate group of PAPS, acts as a catalytic acid to enhance the dissociative nature of the sulphuryl transfer mechanism. The other critical residue is a histidine, which acts as the base which deprotonates the phenol (or other group) to a phenoxide. The resultant nucleophile can then attack the sulphur atom of the transferring sulphuryl group.

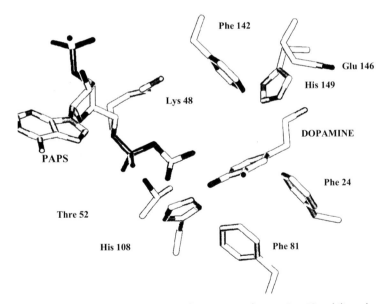

Fig. 7.29 Schematic of he active site of catechol sulpho-transferase (SULT1A3).with dopamine in the active site. Phe 142, 81 and 24 form a hydrophobic pocket, whilst Glu 146 provides an ion-pair interaction with the substrate. Leu 48 stabilises the transition state and His 108 deprotonates one of the catechol hydroxyl groups to form the phenoxide nucleophile to allow the reaction to proceed.

The glucuronide and sulpho-transferases are present in the gut as well as the liver and catalyse the metabolism of many phenol or catechol-containing drugs (morphine, isoprenaline, etc.) during passage through the gut. The ready conjugation of phenolic functions by both glucuronyl and sulpho-transferase systems means that drugs such as morphine are cleared to both glucuronide and sulphate metabolites.

7.7.2
Methyl Transferases

Structural data are available on a third member of the transferases, catechol-methyl transferase. These crystal structure data give further clues on how the transferases metabolise their substrates, particularly with regard to the deprotonation step [33]. This enzyme catalyses the transfer of the methyl group from S-adenosyl-L-methionine (SAM) to one hydroxyl group of catechols. Catechols are occasionally present in drug candidates (e.g. felodopam) but are frequently encountered as metabolites of drugs (e.g. methylenedioxy containing compounds such as zamifenacin and paroxetine). The active site of COMT includes the coenzyme-binding motif and the catalytic site situated in the vicinity of the Mg^{2+} ion. The methyl transfer from SAM to the catechol substrate catalysed by COMT is a direct bimolecular transfer of the methyl group from the sulphur of a-Me-DOPA to the oxygen of the catechol hydroxyl in an S_N2-like transition state. The exact juxtaposition of the substrate to the methyl group is possible because of the binding of the two hydroxyl groups to a Mg^{2+} ion. One hydroxyl of the substrate is surrounded by three positively charged groups inducing it to release its proton to become a negatively charged phenolate ion. These moieties are the Mg^{2+}, the methyl group of SAM and Lys 144. The Mg^{2+} ion in particular probably lowers the pK_a of the hydroxyl group significantly. In contrast, the proton of the other hydroxyl is stabilised by the negatively charged carboxyl group of Glu 199. The ionised hydroxyl makes a direct nucleophilic attack on the electron-deficient methyl of a-Me-DOPA.

7.7.3
Glutathione S-Transferases

Glutathione S-transferases (GSTs) are the most important family of enzymes involved in the metabolism of alkylating compounds and their metabolites. They are a major defence system in deactivating toxic materials within the body. The cytosolic GSTs function as dimeric proteins that are assembled from identical or non-identical subunits. Catalytic diversity for the cytosolic isoenzymes originates from the multiplicity of different homo- and hetero-dimeric forms that collectively metabolise a very broad range of structurally diverse electrophilic substrates, although all are highly specific for the thiol-containing substrate glutathione. Understanding the mechanism is considerably helped by the availability of x-ray crystallography data [34].

Each subunit has an active site that appears as a cleft along the domain interface. Each site can be separated into two distinct functional regions: a hydrophilic G-site for binding the physiological substrate glutathione, and an adjacent hydrophobic H-site for binding structurally diverse electrophilic substrates. Although the active sites of glutathione S-transferases are catalytically independent, the full active site is formed by structural elements from both subunits of the dimer. Residues contributing to binding glutathione at the G-site form a network of specific polar interactions. Of key importance is a hydrogen bond between a conserved G-site tyrosine residue and the glutathione thiol group. This hydrogen bond stabilises the thiolate anion of the active site-bound glutathione. Estimated pK_a values for the bound glutathione are at least two below the pK_a value for glutathione free in aqueous solution. The H-site is formed of clusters of non-polar amino acid side chains, which provide a highly hydrophobic surface, that in the absence of a drug substrate is open to bulk solvent. Binding of substrates to this site has been shown to relate to increased lipophilicity (4-hydroxyalkenes). The actual conjugation reaction, with the thiolate anion acting as a nucleophile proceeds via an S_N2-type mechanism yielding the *deactivated* product.

7.8
Stability to Conjugation Processes

Conjugation with glucuronic acid or sulphate requires a nucleophilic substituent present in the molecule normally a hydroxyl function. In the case of the glucuronyl-transferases this can be phenol, primary, secondary or even tertiary alcohol or carboxylate or in the case of sulpho-transferases normally phenol. In some cases primary alcohols can also form sulphate conjugates. The most *reactive* grouping is the phenol and a simple rule is to eliminate such groupings unless essential for activity. In some cases bioisosteres can be introduced to retain pharmacological activity and overcome conjugation. To act as agonists of the dopamine receptor an H-bond donor group is essential in the correct position on a phenyl ring whose centre is situated 5.1 Å from a protonated nitrogen atom [33]. Figure 7.30 illustrates 7-hydroxy-(amino) tetralin analogues, which are potent agonists.

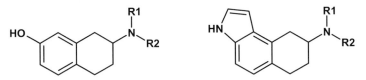

Fig. 7.30 Substitution of a pyrrolo for a phenolic function to act as a H-bond donor for receptor interactions but is resistant to glucuronidation.

These compounds have very low bioavailability and short duration due to extremely rapid glucuronidation [35]. Substitution of the phenolic hydroxy group with a pyrrolo ring gives a compound series with suitable H-bond donor in the correct position (also the geometry matches that of the phenolic hydroxyl), but resistant to glucuronidation [36]. It is not sufficient to replace functionality with groupings with similar chemical properties. For instance tetrazolyl is almost an exact mimic of the carboxyl group and readily undergoes glucuronidation.

Catechol-methyl transferases require the catechol function to be present to bind to the Mg^{2+} ion. In the search for β_2 adrenoceptor selectivity, to produce potent bronchodilators with low cardiovascular effects changing the 3,4-hydroxy grouping of the catechol to 3,5- or 3-hydroxyl, 4-methyl-hydroxy proved important (Fig. 7.31). These compounds now have much improved bioavailability and pharmacokinetics due to their resistance to catechol-methyl transferases.

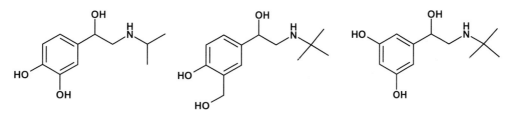

Fig. 7.31 Design of β_2 selective adrenoceptor agonists resistant to catechol-O-methyl transferase (COMT).

7.9
Pharmacodynamics and Conjugation

In a number of cases the transferase enzymes metabolise compounds to active species. Morphine is a highly potent opioid analgesic (Fig. 7.32). It is metabolised by glucuronidation of both its hydroxyl functions by both the gastrointestinal tract and the liver.

Glucuronidation of the 6′-position to form morphine-6-glucuronide gives a compound that is also active [37]. Given systemically, the metabolite is twice as potent as morphine itself. When administered intrathecally the compound is approximately 100-fold more potent than the parent morphine.

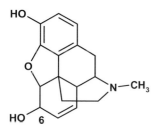

Fig. 7.32 Structure of morphine, which is metabolised to a more active opioid analgesic by glucuronidation at the 6-position.

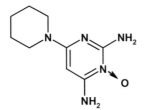

Fig. 7.33 Structure of minoxidil, a compound metabolised by sulpho-transferases to a potassium channel activator.

Unlike morphine, minoxidil [38] is not active itself but is metabolised by hepatic sulpho-transferases to minoxidil N–O sulphate (Fig. 7.33).

Minoxidil sulphate is a potent activator of the ATP-modulated potassium channel and thereby relaxes vascular smooth muscle to give a resultant anti-hypertensive effect. The actual sulphate metabolite is a relatively minor metabolite, the principal metabolite being the N–O glucuronide. The discovery of minoxidil illustrates the caution to be placed on solely *in vitro* screening of compounds. Occasionally *in vivo* experiments will provide significant advances due to metabolism to novel active agents.

References

1 Smith, D.A., Jones, B.C. **1992**, *Biochem. Pharmacol.* 44, 2089–2104.

2 Guengerich, F.P., Hanna, I.H., Martin, M.V., Gillam, E.M.J. **2003**, *Biochem.* 42, 1245–1253.

3 Gillis, A.M., Kates, R.E. **1984**, *Clin. Pharmacokin.* 9, 375–403.

4 Lee, J.T., Kroemer, H.K., Silberstein, D.J., Funck-Brentano, C., Lineberry, M.D., Wood, A.J., Roden, D.M., Woosley, R.L. **1990**, *New England J. Med.* 322, 1764–1768.

5 Manoury, P.M., Binet, J.L., Rousseau, J., Leferre-Borg, F.M., Cavero, I.G. **1987**, *J. Med. Chem.* 30, 1003–1011.

6 Marchetti, P., Natalesi, R. **1989**, *Clin. Pharmacokin.* 16, 100–1286.

7 Verbeck, R.K., Blackburn, J.L., Loewen, G.R. **1983**, *Clin. Pharmacokin.* 8, 297–331.

8 Williams, P.A., Cosme, J., Vinkovi, D.M., Ward, A., Angore, H.C., Day, P.J., Vonrhein, C., Tickle, I.J., Jhoti, H. **2004**, *Science* 305, 683–686.

9 Dugar, S., Yumibe, N., Clader, J.W., Vizziano, M., Huie, K., Heek, M.V., Compton, D.S., Davis, H.R. **1996**, *Biorg. Med. Chem. Lett.* 6, 1271–1274.

10 Penning, T.D., Talley, J.J., Bertenshaw, S.R., Carter, J.S., Collins, P.W., Docter, S., Graneto, M.J., Lee, L.F., Malecha, J.W., Miyashiro, J.M., Rogers, R.S., Rogier, D.J., Yu, S.S., Anderson, G.D., Burton, E.G., Cogburn, E.G., Gregory, S.A., Koboldt, C.M., Perkins, W.E., Seibert, K., Veenhuizen, A.W., Zhang, A.W., Isaakson, P.C. **1997**, *J. Med. Chem.* 40, 1347–1365.

11 Floyd, D.M., Dimball, S.D., Drapcho, J., Das, J., Turk, C.F., Moquin, R.V., Lago, M.W., Duff, K.J., Lee, V.G., White, R.E., Ridgewell, R.E., Moreland, S., Brittain, R.J., Normandin, D.E., Hedberg, S.A., Cucinotta, G.C. **1992**, *J. Med. Chem.* 35, 756–772.

12 Beedham, C. **2002** Molybdenum hydroxylases, in *Enzyme Systems that Metabolise Drugs and Other Xenobiotics*, Ioannides, C. (ed.), Wiley, New York, (pp.) 147–187.

13 Lake, B.G., Ball, S.E., Ka, J., Renwick, A.B., Price, R.J., Scatina, J.A. **2002**, *Xenobiotica* 32, 835–847.

14 Clarke, S.E., Harrell, A.W., Chenery, R.J. **1995**, *Drug Metab. Dispos.* 23, 251–254.

15 Beedham, C., Peet, C.F., Panoutsopou-
lus, G.I., Carter, H., Smith, J.A. **1995**, in
Progress in Brain Research, vol. 106, Yu,
P.M., Tipton, K.F., Boulton, A.A. (ed.),
Elsevier Science BV, Amsterdam, (pp.)
345–353.

16 Macdonald, G.J., Branch, C.K.,
Hadley, M.S., Johnson, C.N., Nash, D.J.,
Smith, A.B., Stemp, G., Thewlis, K.M.,
Vong, A.K.K., Austin, N.E., Jeffrey, P.,
Winborn, K.Y., Boyfield, I., Hagan, J.J.,
Middlemiss, D.N., Reavill, C.,
Riley, G.J., Watson, J.M., Wood, M.,
Parker, S.G., Ashby, R.A. **2003**, *J. Med.
Chem.* 46, 4952–4964.

17 Cashman, J.R. **2003**, *Curr. Opin. Drug
Discov. Devel.* 6, 486–493.

18 Tipton, K.F., Boyce, S., O'Sullivan, J.,
Davey, G.P., Healy, J. **2004**, *Curr. Med.
Chem.* 11, 1965–1982.

19 Benedetti, M.S. **2001**, *Fund. Clin.
Pharm.* 15, 75–84.

20 Dixon, C.M., Park, G., Tarbit, M.H.
1994, *Biochem. Pharmacol.* 47, 1253–
1257.

21 Dixon, C.M., Saynor, D.A.,
Andrew, P.D., Oxford, J., Bradbury, A.,
Tarbit, M.H. **1993**, *Drug Metab. Dispos.*
21, 761–769.

22 Rosenblum, S.B., Huynh, T.,
Afonso, A., Davis, H.R., Yumibe, N.,
Clader, J.W., Burnett, D.A. **1998**, *J. Med.
Chem.* 41, 973–980.

23 Evans, M.E., Stemp, G. **1991**, *Chem.
Brit.* 27, 439–442.

24 Hoke, F., Cunningham, F.,
James, M.K., Muir, K.T., Hoffman, W.E.
1997, *J. Pharmacol. Exp. Ther.* 281, 226–
232.

25 Baxter, A.J., Carr, R.D., Eyley, S.C.,
Fraser-Rae, L., Hallam, C., Harper,
S.T., Hurved, P.A., King, S.J.,

Menchani, P. **1992**, *J. Med. Chem.* 35,
3718–3720.

26 Kumar, G.N., Bodor, N. **1996**, *Curr. Med.
Chem.* 3, 23–36.

27 Kaye, B., Brearley, C.J., Cussans, N.J.,
Herron, M., Humphrey, M.J., Mollatt,
A.R. **1997**, *Xenobiotica* 27, 1091–1102.

28 Burchell, B. **1999** in *Handbook of Drug
Metabolism*, Woolf, T.F. (ed.), Marcel
Dekker, New York, (pp.) 153–173.

29 Yin, H., Bennett, G., Jones, J.P. **1994**,
Chemico Biol. Int. 90, 47–58.

30 Duffel, M.W., Jacoby, W.B. **1981**, *J.Biol.-
Chem.* 256, 11123–11127.

31 Dajani, R., Cleasby, A., Neu, M.,
Wonacott, A.J., Jhoti, H., Hood, A.M.,
Modi, S., Hersey, A., Taskinen, J.,
Cooke, R.M., Manchee, G.R.,
Coughtrie, M.W.H. **1999**, *J. Biol. Chem.*
274, 37862–37868.

32 Kakuta, Y., Petrotchenko, E.V.,
Pedersen, L.C., Negishi, M. **1998**, *J. Biol.
Chem.* 273, 27324–27330.

33 Vidgren, J., Svensson, L.A., Liijas, A.
1994, *Nature* 368, 354–358.

34 Dirr, H., Reinemer, P., Huber, R. **1994**,
Eur. J. Biochem. 220, 645–661.

35 Stjernlof, P., Gullme, M., Elebring, T.,
Anderson, B., Wikstrom, H.,
Lagerquist, S., Svensson, K., Ekman, A.,
Carlsson, A., Sundell, S. **1993**, *J. Med.
Chem.* 36, 2059–2065.

36 Asselin, A.A., Humber, L.G., Roith, K.,
Metcalf, G. **1986**, *J. Med. Chem.* 29, 648–
654.

37 Paul D., Standifer, K.M., Inturrisi, C.E.,
Pasternack, G.W. **1989**, *J. Pharmacol.
Exp. Ther.* 251, 477–483.

38 McCall, J.M., Aiken, J.W.,
Chidester, C.G., DuCharme, D.W.,
Wendling, M.G. **1983**, *J. Med. Chem.* 26,
1791–1793.

8
Toxicity

8.1
Toxicity Findings

A complex series of *in vitro* tests, animal tests and then human exposure can at any stage reveal adverse findings that can be termed toxicity. Broadly, toxicity findings can be broken down into three subdivisions:

8.1.1
Pharmacophore-induced Toxicity

This involves findings relating to the pharmacology of the compound. Within this category the adverse effects are a direct extension of the pharmacology, or an indirect extension. With the indirect extension the original selectivity of the compound for a target is lost at elevated doses and the effects seen are triggered by effects on proteins, etc., closely related structurally to the original target. Pharmacophore-induced toxicity is usually seen at doses in excess of the therapeutic dose.

Pharmacophore-induced toxicity does not necessarily occur within the organ or site of intended therapy. An example of this is the toxicity of loop diuretics [1]. The target for this class of drugs are the Na-(K)-Cl co-transporters of the kidney. These co-transporters play a major role in the ion transport and fluid secretion of the utricle and semicircular canal of the ear. Perhaps not surprisingly loop diuretics are associated with ototoxicity. The selectivity and potency of various diuretics can explain their different toxicity profile. Kidney-specific co-transporters ENCC1 and ENCC2 are expressed in the thick ascending limb and distal convoluted tubule, respectively. ENCC3 is expressed in many tissues including the cochlea. Thiazide diuretics only have activity against ENCC1 and show no toxicity. Loop diuretics inhibit NKCC2 with potencies for bumetanide $< 0.2\,\mu M$ and NKCC3 $> 0.5\,\mu M$. The selectivity of the compound for NKCC2 is lost under the conditions which cause the ototoxicity: intravenous administration of high doses.

Pharmacokinetics and Metabolism in Drug Design.
Dennis A. Smith, Han van de Waterbeemd, Don K. Walker (Eds.)
Copyright © 2006 WILEY-VCH Verlag GmbH & Co. KGaA, Weinheim
ISBN: 3-527-31368-0

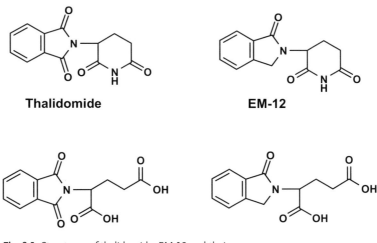

Thalidomide   **EM-12**

Fig. 8.1 Structures of thalidomide, EM-12 and their metabolites which are all angiogenesis inhibitors and teratogens or potential teratogens.

Unexpected or polypharmacology in a structure can occasionally lead to additional benefits in drugs. In the same way polypharmacology can have dramatic consequences in toxicity. Thalidomide was used as an anti-nauseant to control morning sickness. Its use in pregnant women had terrible consequences due to the teratogenic nature of the drug.

Recently thalidomide and some of its metabolites (Fig. 8.1) and related analogues have been shown to be inhibitors [2] of hFGF and VEGF-induced neovascularisation (angiogenesis). Such a finding readily provides a hypothesis since limb development (the site of teratogenesis) is dependant on the formation of new blood vessels.

A problem with toxicity produced by an extension of the compounds pharmacology is that the conventional use of no-effect doses based on pre-clinical animal studies may not apply. Moreover, pre-clinical studies may be complicated in the often understated ranges of response seen across species due to species differences in the receptors, enzymes and ion channels that compromise drug targets. Table 8.1 lists some of these known variations and the consequences range from an exaggerated response, to an absence of a response.

Tab. 8.1 Receptors, ion channels and enzymes which are drug
targets and show species differences.

Receptors

Adenosine	A_1, A_2	Luteinizing hormone	LH
Adrenoceptors	a_{1B}, a_{1C}, a_{2A}	Muscarinic	M_2
Atrial natriuretic factor	ANF-R1	Neurokinin	NK_1, NK_3
Bradykinin	B_2	Purinoceptors	P_2
Cholecystokinin	CCK	Thromboxane	TA_2
Dopamine	D_1	Vanilloid	
Endothelin	ET_B	Vasopressin	V_1
Serotonin	$5\text{-HT}_{1A, B, D}$ $5\text{-HT}_2, 5\text{-HT}_3, 5\text{-HT}_4$		

Ion channels

Rapidly activating delayed
rectifier K^+ channel

Enzymes

Carbopeptidase B	Renin
Na^+/K^+ ATPase	HMG-CoA reductase

8.1.2
Structure-related Toxicity

Findings related to the structure of the compound but not related to the pharmacology. This category is distinguished by the adverse events or effects being triggered by structural features or physicochemical properties, etc., which allow the compound or metabolites to interact at sites distinct from the intended target or related proteins, etc. This type of toxicity can occur at any dose level including the therapeutic dose.

Amiodarone (Fig. 8.2) is an efficacious drug that causes a number of side effects. The presence of iodine in the molecule is unusual. Hypothyroidism and hyperthyroidism have been reported in patients. Although the loss of iodine is relatively slow, the relatively large daily dose size and long half-life of the drug and its de-ethylated metabolite suggest that the presence of iodine in the molecule is responsible for this toxicity [3].

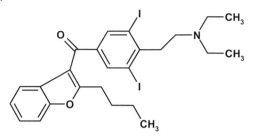

Fig. 8.2 Structure of the highly lipophilic anti-arrhythmic, amiodarone.

The drug is also a highly lipophilic base and accumulates in a number of tissues including the lung. This combination of extreme physicochemical properties can result in more specific interactions such as the condition of phospholipidosis (increase in total lung phospholipids) caused by inhibition of phospholipid break-down [4]. The medicinal chemist has to decide if extreme lipophilicity and the presence of iodine are essential for activity, and in the case of amiodarone, have proven clinical efficacy or whether alternative structures are possible.

Proxicromil and FPL 52757 [5] were oral anti-allergy agents that utilised the strongly acidic *chromone* skeleton as a starting point (Fig. 8.3). This skeleton contained the pharmacophore. To achieve oral absorption substantial lipophilicity was added and these changes resulted in surface-active (detergent) molecules. The hepatobiliary route of excretion and resultant high concentrations of the compounds at the biliary canaliculus resulted in hepatotoxicity [5].

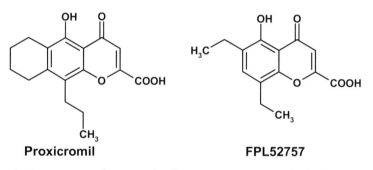

Proxicromil **FPL52757**

Fig. 8.3 Structures of proxicromil and FPL52757, two compounds which exhibited toxicity due to physicochemical properties.

8.1.3
Metabolism-induced Toxicity

Metabolism-induced toxicity is where a key function or grouping is altered by oxidation, reduction or conjugation to become reactive, normally an electrophile [6]. The electrophilic group is then capable of reacting with nucleophiles in the body. Nucleophilic functions are present in proteins, nucleic acids and small peptides such as glutathione. Reactions with these targets can lead to organ toxicity including carcinogenesis or simply excretion from the body (glutathione conjugates). Some indication of possible target [7] is indicated by the nature of the electrophile produced (soft-hard), as indicated in Fig. 8.4.

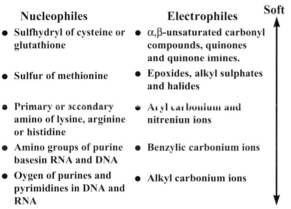

Fig. 8.4 Schematic showing relative softness and hardness of nucleophiles and electrophiles as an indicator of sites of reaction of electrophilic metabolites.

Compounds that react with amino acids or proteins can trigger toxicity by two mechanisms. The direct mechanism involves reaction with specific proteins and altering their function such that cell death and necrosis occurs. Such toxicities are often seen in a large number of subjects and are dose related. They are also often predictable by animal studies. Alternative mechanisms of toxicity involve an immune component, whereby the protein-metabolite conjugate triggers an immune response. Such toxicity is termed idiosyncratic, occurring in only a subset of the patients receiving the drug. This type of toxicity is not predicted normally by animal studies. These two types of toxicity are illustrated in the schematic shown in Fig. 8.5. Glutathione and the glutathione transferase enzymes protect the body from the reactive metabolites. This system is saturable, so that a threshold dose, or other factors leading to glutathione depletion, is needed to trigger the toxicity.

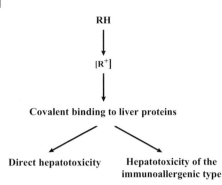

Fig. 8.5 Schematic showing the generation of a reactive metabolite, its reaction with a protein target, and toxicity being exerted by a direct mechanism (protein essential to cell function) or one involving the immune system.

8.2
Importance of Dose Size

Regardless of the specific toxicity, the impact of administered dose should not be underestimated. For an oral drug the dose size gives a measure of the insult to the gastrointestinal tract, the fraction that is absorbed representing the insult to liver and the concentration of drug (and possibly metabolites) in the systemic circulation or individual organs the insult to the rest of the body. Special consideration in post-hepatic fate needs to be placed on the kidney due to its ability to transport and concentrate intracellularly drug and metabolites. Table 8.2 lists drugs withdrawn from the market over the last 30 years due to hepatotoxicity. The drugs include a number of different drug classes and have very divergent structures. It is noticeable that most of the drugs have high to very high clinical doses. This makes no assumptions about mechanism/structure, etc., but indicates that toxicity is related to mass and hence the normal principles of chemical thermodynamics. The importance of dose size will be further emphasised in Section 8.14.

8.3
Epoxides

Epoxide metabolites can be generated from a variety of aromatic systems. Anticonvulsants are a class of drug whose side effects, such as hepatic necrosis and aplastic anaemia, are thought to be mediated by chemically reactive epoxide metabolites formed by cytochrome P450 oxidation. For instance phenytoin (Fig. 8.6) toxicity is correlated with oxidation and the inhibition of epoxide hydrolase [8].

Tab. 8.2 Drugs withdrawn since 1960 due to hepatotoxicity and their daily clinical dose.

Generic name	Dose (mg)
Isaxonine	1500
Fenclofenac	1200
Nitrefazole	1200
Ebrotidine	800
Pirprofen	800
Benoxaprofen	600
Chlormezanon	600
Flipexide	600
Ibufenac	600
Suloctidyl	600
Bendazac	500
Moxisylyte	480
Clometacin	450
Tienilic acid	400
Troglitazone	400
Tolrestat	400
Fenclozic acid	400
Perhexiline	400
Tolcapone	300
Zimeldine	300
Cyclofenil	200
Dilevalol	200
Trovafloxicin	200
Exifone	180
Pemoline	180
Nomifensine	125
Nialamide	100
Mebanazine	30

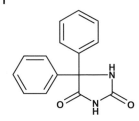

Fig. 8.6 Structure of phenytoin, a drug believed to exert its toxicity through reactive epoxide metabolites.

Carbamazepine exerts its anti-convulsant activity through its own action on voltage sensitive sodium channels and those of its relatively stable 10-11-epoxide. The compound shows a number of potential toxicities including skin rash, hepatic necrosis and teratogenicity. It is possible the 10-11-epoxide is the causative agent but structural studies [9] suggest other epoxide metabolites of the aromatic ring may be responsible in part. Oxcarbazepine (Fig. 8.7) is a related drug that cannot form the 10-11-epoxide and also owes part of its activity to a metabolite (hydroxyl). Oxcarbazepine is much less teratogenic in animal models and shows a lower preponderance of skin rash [8, 10].

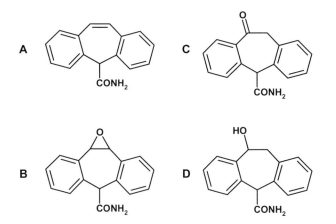

Fig. 8.7 Structures of carbamazepine (A), its 10-11-epoxide metabolite (B), and oxcarbazepine (C) and its hydroxyl metabolite (D).

8.4
Quinone Imines

Phenacetin is a classical example of this with oxidation of the compound by cytochrome P450 leading to a benzoquinone intermediate (Fig. 8.8). The benzoquinone reacts with various cytosolic proteins to trigger a direct hepatotoxicity [6].

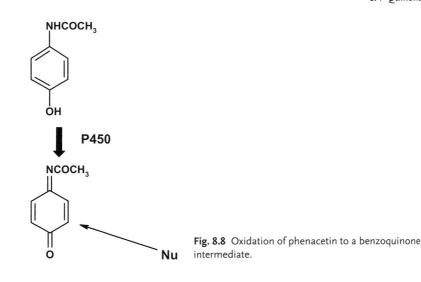

Fig. 8.8 Oxidation of phenacetin to a benzoquinone intermediate.

Toxicity by metabolism is not confined to the liver since oxidative systems occur in many organs and cells. Amodiaquine is a 4-aminoquinoline anti-malarial that has been associated with hepatitis and agranulocytosis. Both side effects are probably triggered by reactive metabolites produced in the liver or in other sites of the body. For instance polymorphonuclear leucocytes can oxidise amodiaquine. The same pathway to a quinone imine is implicated (Fig. 8.9) to that seen for acetaminophen [11] indicating the advisability to avoid such structural features in a molecule.

Such reactions can occur in other molecules containing aromatic amine functions without a para-oxygen substituent. For instance diclofenac can be oxidised to a minor metabolite (5-OH) diclofenac, which can be further oxidised [12] to the benzoquinine imine metabolite (Fig. 8.10).

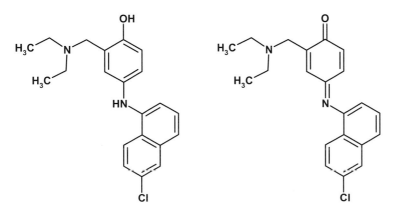

Fig. 8.9 Structures of amodiaquine and its quinone imine metabolite.

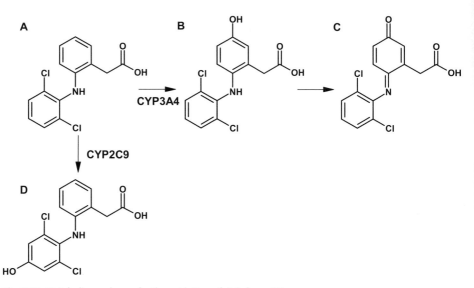

Fig. 8.10 Metabolism scheme for the oxidation of diclofenac (A) to benzoquinone imine (C) metabolites.

Again, the reactivity of this intermediate has been implicated in the hepatotoxicity of the compound.

Another drug with a high incidence of hepatotoxicity is the acetylcholinesterase inhibitor tacrine. Binding of reactive metabolites to liver tissue correlated with the formation of a 7-hydroxy metabolite [13], highly suggestive of a quinone imine metabolite as the reactive species. Such a metabolite would be formed by further oxidation of 7-hydroxy tacrine (Fig. 8.11).

Indomethacin, is associated, in the clinic, with a relatively high incidence of agranulocytosis. Although indomethacin itself is not oxidised to reactive metabolites, one of its metabolites, desmethyldeschlorobenzoylindomethacin (DMBI)

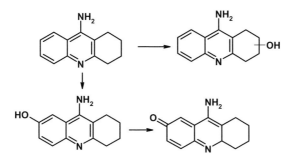

Fig. 8.11 Metabolism of tacrine to hydroxyl metabolites, the 5-hydroxy derivative of which can be further oxidised to the reactive quinone imine.

forms an iminoquinone [14]. Formation of the iminoquinone from DMBI is cata-lysed by myeloperoxidase (the major oxidising enzyme in neutrophils) and HOCl (the major oxidant produced by activated neutrophils). The pathway for formation of the iminoquinone is illustrated in Fig. 8.12.

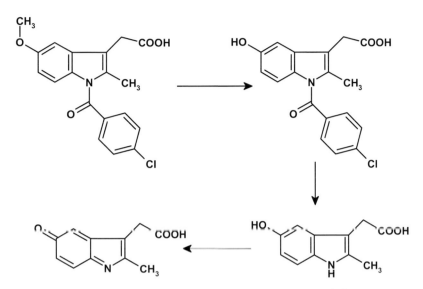

Fig. 8.12 Metabolism of indomethacin to a reactive iminoquinone metabolite.

Practolol (Fig. 8.13) was the prototype cardioselective β-adrenoceptor blocking agent. The selectivity was obtained by substitution in the para-position with an acetyl anilino function. The similarity of this drug with those outlined above is obvious. Practolol caused severe skin and eye lesions in some patients that led to its withdrawal from the market [6]. These lesions manifested as a rash, hyperkera-

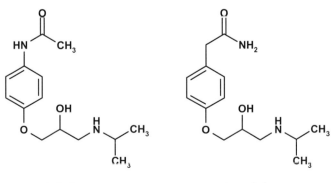

practolol   atenolol

Fig. 8.13 Structures of practolol and atenolol.

tosis, scarring, even perforation of the cornea and development of fibrovascular mass in the conjunctiva, and sclerosing peritonitis. Some evidence is available that the drug is oxidatively metabolised to a reactive product that binds irreversibly to tissue proteins.

That the toxic functionality is the acetanilide is confirmed by the safety of a follow-up drug atenolol. Atenolol (Fig. 8.13) has identical physicochemical properties and a very similar structure except that the acetyl-amino function has been replaced with an amide grouping. This structure cannot give rise to similar aromatic amine reactive metabolites.

The withdrawal of practolol from the market place is obviously a severe step for the company and those patients benefiting. Although not shown to be causative the presence of an aromatic amine in the structure of nomifensine (Fig. 8.14) has to be treated with suspicion, the compound was also withdrawn from the market nine years after launch due to a rising incidence of acute immune haemolytic anaemia [15].

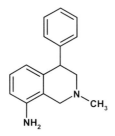

Fig. 8.14 Structure of nomifensine, an anti-depressant associated with acute immune haemolytic anaemia.

Carbutamide was the first oral anti-diabetic, and the prototype for the sulphonamide type of agent. Carbutamide caused marked bone marrow toxicity in man, but derivatives of this, not containing the anilino function, such as tolbutamide (Fig. 8.15), were devoid of such toxicity. As for many of the agents featured in this

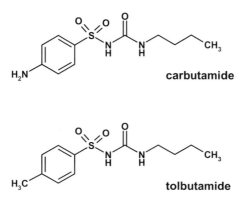

carbutamide

tolbutamide

Fig. 8.15 Structures of carbutamide an oral anti-diabetic, associated with bone marrow toxicity, and tolbutamide a compound, devoid of similar findings.

section the structural similarity between carbutamide and tolbutamide clearly implicates the anilino function as the toxicophore.

A further example of the design of drugs to remove aromatic amine functionality even when present as a amide is illustrated by the Na^+ channel class of anti-arrhythmic drugs [16]. Lidocaine is very rapidly metabolised (Fig. 8.16) so is only useful as a short-term intravenous agent. Oral forms include procainamide, tocainide and flecainide (Fig. 8.16). Procainamide causes fatal bone marrow aplasia in 0.2% of patients and lupus syndrome in 25–50%. Tocainide also causes bone marrow aplasia and pulmonary fibrosis. In contrast, flecainide, whose structure contains no aromatic amine, masked or otherwise, has adverse effects related directly to its pharmacology. Interestingly, the lupus syndrome seen with procainamide is largely absent when N-acetyl procainamide is substituted.

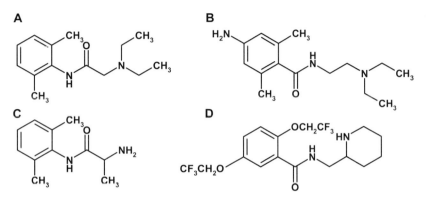

Fig. 8.16 Structures of Na^+ channel blocker anti-arrythmics: lidocaine (A), procaineamide (B), tocainide (C) and flecainide (D).

8.5
Nitrenium Ions

Clozapine, an anti-psychotic agent, has the potential to cause agranulocytosis with an incidence of 1%. The major oxidant in human neutrophils, HOCl, oxidises clozapine to a nitrenium ion (Fig. 8.17) in which the positive charge is highly delocalised. This metabolite is capable of binding irreversibly to the neutrophil [17]. A variety of cells including liver, neutrophils and bone marrow can form reactive clozapine metabolites that react to form glutathione thioether adducts [18].

Various analogues have been investigated indicating that the nitrogen-bridge between the two aromatic rings is the target at least for HOCl oxidation. When alternative bridging heteroatoms are used (Fig. 8.18), similar reactive metabolites are not observed [19].

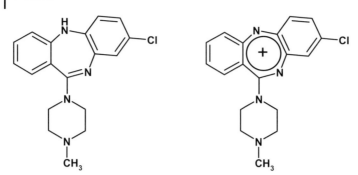

Fig. 8.17 Structures of clozapine and its nitrenium ion, the postulated reactive metabolite generated by oxidation.

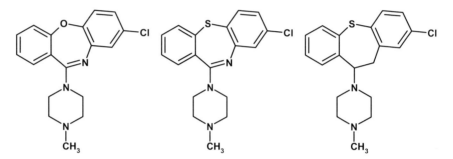

Fig. 8.18 Alternative structures which will not generate the nitrenium ion observed with clozapine.

8.6
Iminium Ions

Mianserin is a tetracyclic anti-depressant that causes agranulocytosis in isolated cases in patients. Detailed structural analysis [20] has indicated that oxidation by cytochrome P450 to one or more iminium ions is the likely first step in this toxicity, the most likely being the C4-N5 version (Fig. 8.19). Evidence for this is provided by the C14β methyl and the O10 analogues which cannot form the corresponding nitrenium and carbonium ions, but are cytotoxic. Removal of the N5-nitrogen atom in analogous structures abolishes production of the reactive metabolites (Fig. 8.20).

Vesnarinone is a drug for congestive heart failure associated with a 1% incidence of agranulocytosis. When metabolised by activated neutrophils the major metabolite is vertrylpiperazinamide (Fig. 8.21). This unusual N-dealkylation (of an aromatic ring) can be rationalised by chlorination of the nitrogen, to which the aromatic ring is attached by HOCl, followed by loss of HCl to form the reactive iminium ion, which itself can react with nucleophiles. Hydrolysis of the iminium ion yields vertrylpiperazinamide and another reactive species, the quinone imine (see Section 8.4).

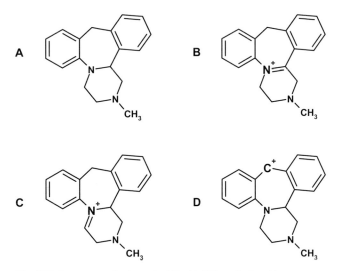

Fig. 8.19 Structures of mianserin (A) with N5 marked and its
putative reactive metabolites: N5-C14β iminium ion (B),
C4-N5 iminium ion (C) and carbonium ion at C10 (D).
Evidence indicates metabolite B as the causative agent.

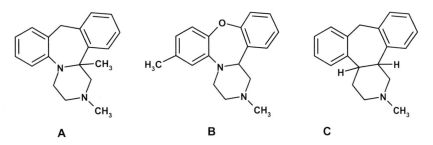

Fig. 8.20 Structures of mianserin analogues. A and B cannot
form the N5-C14β iminium C10 carbonium ion but are still toxic.
C without the N5 nitrogen is not toxic implicating the
C4-N5 imminium ion.

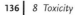

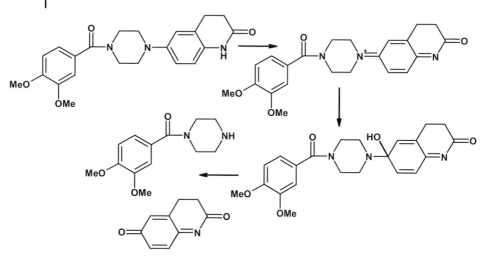

Fig. 8.21 Structures of vesnarinone, and its major metabolite vertrylpiperazinamide. The pathway metabolised by activated neutrophils gives rise to two highly reactive species, an imminium ion and a quinone imine.

8.7
Hydroxylamines

Sulfonamide anti-microbial agents (Fig. 8.22) such as sulfamethoxazole [21] are oxidised to protein-reactive cytotoxic metabolites in the liver and also other tissues. These include hydroxylamines and further products such as nitroso-derivatives. Sulfonamide drugs are linked with agranulocytosis, aplastic anaemia, skin and mucous membrane hypersensitivity reactions including Stevens–Johnson, etc. Dapsone [22] is a potent anti-inflammatory and anti-parasitic compound, which is metabolised by cytochrome P450 to hydroxylamines, which in turn cause methemoglobinemia and hemolysis.

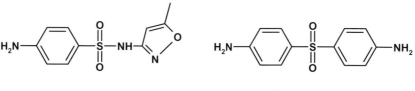

Sulphamethoxazole　　　　　　　　　　**Dapsone**

Fig. 8.22 Structures of sulfamethoxazole and dapsone, drugs which form toxic hydroxylamine metabolites.

8.8
Thiophene Rings

Thiophene rings are another functionality that are easily activated to electrophilic species. Thiophene itself is metabolised to the S-oxide, which is viewed as the key primary reactive intermediate. Nucleophilic groups such as thiols react at position 2 of the thiophene S-oxide via a Michael-type addition [23]. Tienilic acid (Fig. 8.23) is oxidised to an S-oxide metabolite [24]. This creates two electron-withdrawing substituents on C2 and a resultant strongly electrophilic carbon at C5 of the thiophene ring [24]. This highly reactive metabolite covalently binds to the enzyme metabolising it (CYP2C9), triggering an autoimmune reaction resulting in hepatitis. Rotation of the thiophene ring leads to a compound in which the sulphoxide is less reactive and can create a less reactive sulphoxide metabolite, which reacts primarily at C2 with nucleophiles [24]. This metabolite is stable enough to escape the enzyme and alkylate other proteins leading to direct toxicity.

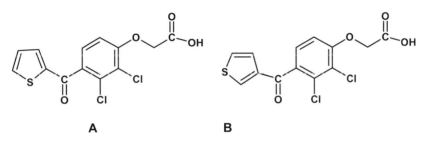

A **B**

Fig. 8.23 Structure of tienilic acid (A) and an isomeric variant (B) which cause hepatotoxicity by autoimmune and direct mechanisms, respectively, following conversion to sulphoxide metabolites and resultant electrophilic carbon atoms.

The thiophene ring has also been incorporated into a number of drugs that have some diverse toxicities associated with them (Fig. 8.24). Ticlodipine, a platelet function inhibitor is associated with agranulocytosis in patients [25]. Suprofen, a non-steroidal anti-inflammatory agent has been withdrawn from the market due to acute renal injury [26].

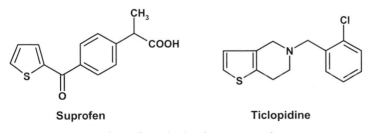

Suprofen **Ticlopidine**

Fig. 8.24 Structures of suprofen and ticlopidine, compounds containing a thiophene ring and associated with diverse toxicities in patients.

The association of ticlodipine with agranulocytosis has been further investigated [27]. A general hypothesis for white blood cell toxicity is activation of the drug to a reactive metabolite by HOCl, the principal oxidant generated by activated neutrophils and monocytes (as in Section 8.4). Under these types of oxidation conditions, ticlodipine is activated to a thiophene-S-chloride (Fig. 8.25), which reacts further to form other products including a glutathione conjugate.

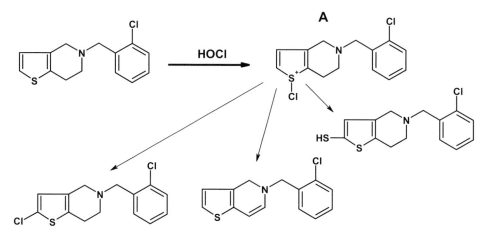

Fig. 8.25 Metabolism of ticlopidine to the reactive thiophene-S-chloride (A) by white blood cells and further breakdown products of this reactive metabolite.

Tenidap (Fig. 8.26) is a dual cyclooxygenase (COX) and 5-lipoxygenase (5-LPO) inhibitor, developed as an anti-inflammatory agent. Severe abnormalities in hepatic function were reported in Japanese clinical trials [28]. Although the thiophene is not directly implicated in these findings, the ready activation of this system to potential reactive metabolites may be suggestive of this function's involvement.

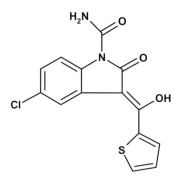

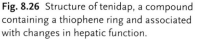

Fig. 8.26 Structure of tenidap, a compound containing a thiophene ring and associated with changes in hepatic function.

8.9
Thioureas

The thiourea group has been incorporated in a number of drugs. The adverse reactions of such compounds are associated with the thiocarbonyl moiety. The thiocarbonyl moiety can be metabolised by flavin-containing mono-oxygenases and cytochrome P450 enzymes to reactive sulfenic, sulfinic and sulfonic acids, which can alkylate proteins. The prototype H_2 antagonist metiamide [29] incorporated a thiourea group. This compound caused blood dyscrasias in man. Replacement of the thiourea [29] with a cyanimino grouping produced the very successful compound cimetidine (Fig. 8.27).

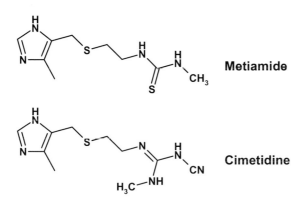

Fig. 8.27 Structures of the thiourea containing H_2 antagonist metiamide, which caused blood dyscrasias in man, and its cyanoimino containing analogue cimetidine which did not show similar adverse findings.

8.10
Chloroquinolines

Chloroquinolines are reactive groupings due to an electron-deficient carbon to which the halogen is attached. This carbon is electron-deficient due to the combined electron withdrawing effects of the chlorine substituent and the quinoline nitrogen. The electrophilic carbon is thus able to react readily with nucleophiles present in the body. The impact of this grouping on a molecule is illustrated by 6-chloro-4-oxo-10-propyl-4H-pyrano[3,2-g]quinoline-2,8-dicarboxylate (Fig. 8.28). In contrast to many related compounds (chromone-carboxylates) lacking the chloroquinoline, 6-chloro-4-oxo-10-propyl-4H-pyrano[3,2-g]quinoline-2,8-dicarboxylate is excreted as a glutathione conjugate [30] formed by nucleophilic attack on the halogen of the chloroquinoline function by the thiol group of glutathione and resultant halogen displacement. Other compounds are excreted as unchanged drugs with no evidence for any metabolism. Moreover, the reactivity of the chloroquino-

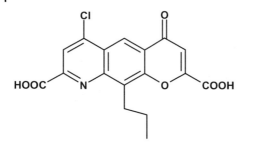

Fig. 8.28 Structure of 6-chloro-4-oxo-10-propyl-4*H*-pyrano [3,2-g]quinoline-2,8-dicarboxylate which, in contrast, to many related compounds (chromone-carboxylates) lacking the chloroquinoline, is excreted as a glutathione conjugate.

line is illustrated by the observation that the reaction with glutathione occurs without enzyme (glutathione S-transferase) present *in vitro*, albeit at a slower rate.

8.11
Stratification of Toxicity

Table 8.3 gives a summary of the various toxicities and the stages at which they can occur. Also summarised is the cause and reasons for the specificity of the effect. With mutagenicity, certain pre-clinical toxicity, carcinogenicity and late clinical toxicology the actual structure of the molecule is important and care should be taken to avoid the incorporation of toxicophores as outlined above. Direct toxicity is addressed by ensuring the daily dose size is low, the intrinsic selectivity high and physicochemical properties within reasonable boundaries.

Tab. 8.3 Various expressions of toxicity and their cause relating to the stage of drug development.

Mutagenicity	Metabolites react with nucleic acid.	Metabolites sufficiently stable to cross nuclear membrane.
Pre-clinical and early clinical	Direct toxicity related to dose size and intrinsic selectivity. Metabolites react with protein and cause cell death.	Over-stimulation of receptor and others in superfamily. Metabolites not detoxified by glutathione, etc.
Carcinogenicity	Metabolites react with nucleic acid or hormonal effects	Metabolites not detoxified by glutathione, etc. Effects on thyroxine, etc., drives pituitary tumors.
Late clinical	Metabolites react with protein	Protein adduct acts as immunogen; immune response involved in toxicity.

8.12
Toxicity Prediction: Computational Toxicology

With increasing toxicity data of various kinds, more reliable predictions based on structure–toxicity relationships of toxic endpoints can be attempted [31–36]. Even the Internet can be used as a source for toxicity data, be it with caution [37]. A number of predictive methods have been compared from a regulatory perspective [35]. Often traditional QSAR approaches using multiple linear regression are used [38]. Newer approaches include the use of neural networks in structure–toxicity relationships [39]. An expert system such as DEREK is yet another approach. Attempts have been made to integrate physiologically-based pharmacokinetic/pharmacodynamic (PBPK/PD) and quantitative structure–activity relationship (QSAR) modelling in toxicity prediction [40]. Most methods need further developments [41]. Currently these approaches can serve to give a first alert, rather than be truly predictive. But also, animal models are not perfect and fully predictive. By comparing animal models to human data of 131 pharmaceutical agents, a true positive prediction of rate of animal models for human toxicity of 69% was observed [42].

New technologies are based on advances in understanding and analysing the effects of chemicals on gene expression or protein expression and processing [43, 44]. More developments can be expected in the coming years.

8.13
Toxicogenomics

A new subdiscipline derived from a combination of the fields of toxicology and genomics is termed toxicogenomics [45]. Using genomics resources, its aim is to study the potential toxic effects of drugs and environmental toxicants. DNA microarrays or *chips* are now available to monitor the expression levels of thousands of genes simultaneously as a marker for toxicity. The complexity of the microarrays yield almost too much data. For instance, initial comparisons of the expression patterns for 100 toxic compounds, using all genes on a DNA microarray failed to discriminate between cytotoxic anti-inflammatory drugs and DNA-damaging agents [46]. A major obstacle encountered in these studies was the lack of reproducible gene responses, presumably due to biological variability and technological limitations. Thus multiple replicated observations for the prototypical DNA-damaging agent, cisplatin, and the non-steroidal anti-inflammatory drugs (NSAIDs) diflunisal and flufenamic acid were made, and a subset of genes yielding reproducible inductions/repressions was selected for comparison. Many of the *fingerprint genes* identified in these studies were consistent with previous observations reported in the literature (e.g. the well-characterised induction by cisplatin of p53-regulated transcripts such as p21waf1/cip1 and PCNA (proliferating cell nuclear antigen)). These gene subsets not only discriminated among the three compounds in the learning set, but also showed predictive value for the rest of the database (ca. 100 compounds of various toxic mechanisms). Further refinement of the clustering strategy, yielded even better results and demonstrated that genes that ultimately best discriminated between DNA damage and NSAIDs were involved in such diverse processes as DNA repair, xenobiotic metabolism, transcriptional activation, structural maintenance, cell cycle control, signal transduction, and apoptosis. The genes span the cycle a cell will go through from initial insult to repair response; further understanding of these cycles will not only allow very sensitive assays for toxicants, but also greater understanding of the molecular events of toxicity.

One even more focussed direction of this work is to explore the pathway resulting from oxidative stress. Exposure of cells to toxic chemicals can result in reduced glutathione (GSH) depletion, generation of free radicals, and binding to critical cell constituents. This binding and resultant chemical stress is usually followed by a concerted cellular response aimed at restoring homeostasis, although the precise initial stimulus for the response is unclear. One component of this stress response is the up-regulation of γ-glutamylcysteine synthetase (γ-GCS) and the preceding molecular events involved in its regulation. C-jun and c-fos mRNA (mRNA) levels and activator protein 1 (AP-1) have been found to be sensitive markers for a number of toxicants [47].

8.14
Enzyme Induction (CYP3A4) and Drug Design

Although largely an adaptive response and not a toxicity, enzyme induction, in particular cytochrome P450, is an undesirable drug interaction, effecting the efficacy of a drug or co-administered drugs. The number of clinically used drugs which induce P450 enzymes is, in fact, quite limited. However, in certain disease areas (AIDS, epilepsy) many of the drugs used, whether for primary or secondary indications, have the potential for enzyme induction. Induction is often seen preclinically, due to the elevated dose levels used, but this potential rarely transfers to the clinical situation [46].

No clear SAR emerges for induction, nor are any particular groups or functions implicated as shown by the diverse structures of the known CYP3A4 inducers (Fig. 8.29). Structures are diverse but most are lipophilic as defined by a positive calculated log P value.

A critical factor in P450 induction in the clinic, based on the known drugs, is dose size. The major inducible form of P450 in man is CYP3A4. The drugs that induce CYP3A4 are given in high doses, often around 500–1000 mg day^{-1} (Table 8.4). These result in total drug concentrations in the 10–100 µM range, or approximately an order of magnitude lower than expressed as a free drug concentration (Table 8.4). The concentrations equate closely to the therapeutic plasma concentrations presented in Table 8.4. These data both reflect the relatively weak affinity of the inducing agents and the need for high concentrations or doses. The high clinical concentrations reflect the weak potency of the drugs. For instance, the Na$^+$

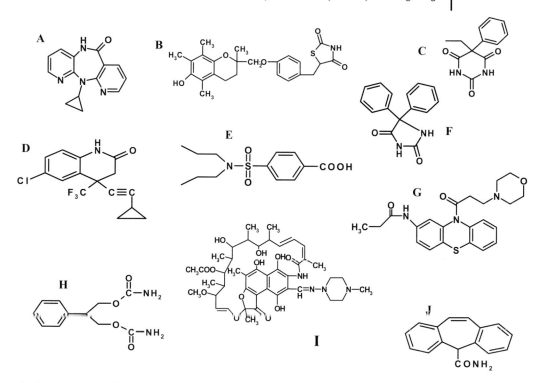

Fig. 8.29 Structures of known clinical CYP3A4 inducers: nevirapine (A), troglitazone (B), phenobarbitone (C), efavirenz (D), probenicid (E), phenytoin (F), moricizine (G), felbamate (H), rifampicin (I), carbamazepine (J).

channel blockers have affinities of 3, 9 and 25 μM (moricizine, phenytoin and carbamazepine, respectively). With the anti-infectives there is the need to dose to IC_{95} or greater. Thus, although efavirenz is a potent inhibitor of wild type RT HIV (K_i of 3 nM), there is a need to go to higher concentrations to reach the IC_{95} for the virus and also to treat for possible mutants.

In contrast to these concentrations many clinically-used drugs, which are non-inducers, are effective at doses up to two orders of magnitude lower. The need for high doses has other undesirable complications. As outlined above, dose size is important in toxicity and enzyme inducers show a high level of adverse drug reactions affecting such organs and tissues as the liver, blood and skin (Table 8.5).

This statement is somewhat at odds with the conventional view that idiosyncratic toxicology is dose size-independent. Idiosyncratic reactions are thought to result from an immune-mediated cell injury triggered by previous contact with the drug. The toxicity may appear after several asymptomatic administrations of the compound (sensitization period) and is not perceived as dose-dependent. For instance, when the relationship between the occurrence of adverse side effects and the use of anti-epileptic drugs were examined there was no definite dose or

Tab. 8.4 Dose, total and free plasma concentrations for clinical CYP3A4 inducers.

	Dose (mg day^{-1})	C_p (µM)	C_p free (µM)
Carbamazepine	400–1200	12	3.6
Phenytoin	350–1000	54	5
Rifampicin	450–600	12	4
Phenobarbitone	70–400	64	32
Troglitazone	200–600	7	0.01
Efavirenz	600	29	0.3
Nevirapine	400	31	12
Moricizine	100–400	3	0.5
Probenicid	1000–2000	350	35
Felbamate	1200–3600	125	95

Tab. 8.5 Clinical toxicities and side effects of P4503A4 inducers.

Carbamazepine	**Aplastic anaemia, agranulocytosis, skin rash, hepatitis**
Phenytoin	Agranulocytosis, skin rash, hepatitis
Rifampicin	Shock, hemolytic anaemia, renal failure.
Phenobarbitone	Aplastic anaemia, agranulocytosis, skin rash
Troglitazone	Hepatic toxicity
Efavirenz	Hepatitis, skin rash
Nevirapine	Hepatitis, skin rash
Moricizine	Prodysrhythmia
Probenicid	Aplastic anaemia, hepatic necrosis
Felbamate	Aplastic anaemia

serum concentration-dependent increase. In fact on closer examination idiosyncratic toxicology and dose size seem firmly linked. Not in the terms of a single drug used over its clinical dose range as above, but that adverse reactions occur more often with high dose drugs. Aside from the examples above an excellent example is clozapine and its close structural analogue olanzapine (Fig. 8.30). Clozapine is used clinically over the dose range of 150–450 mg and its use is associated with agranulocytosis. Olanzipine is used clinically at 5–10 mg and has a

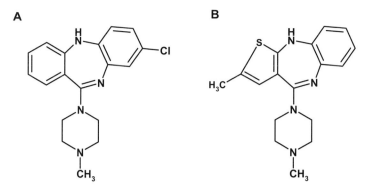

Fig. 8.30 Structures of clozapine (A) and olanzapine (B).

negligible risk from this toxicity. As outlined in Section 8.4, both compounds could potentially be activated to reactive intermediates such as nitrenium ions.

The impact of reducing dose size by either intrinsic potency increases or optimising pharmacokinetics is also critical to avoiding P450 induction. An example of this is the anti-diabetic compound troglitazone (Fig. 8.31). This is used at a relatively high clinical dose (Table 8.4) and its use is associated with enzyme induction. For instance troglitazone lowers the plasma concentrations of known CYP3A4 substrates such as cyclosporine, terfenadine, atorvastatin, and ethinylestradiol. In contrast, the structurally related rosiglitazone (Fig. 8.31) is administered at a lower dose and shows no evidence of enzyme induction. Concomitant administration of rosiglitazone (8 mg) did not effect the pharmacokinetics of the CYP 3A4 substrates nifedipine or ethinylestradiol. The clinical dose used closely relates to the receptor potency of these agents. For instance the EC_{50} values for troglitazone and rosiglitazone for affinity against the peroxisome proliferator-activated receptor γ (PPAR-γ) ligand binding domain are 322 nM and 36 nM, respectively. Corresponding figures for elevation of P2 mRNA levels as a result of peroxisome proliferator-activated receptor γ agonism are 690 and 80 nM, respectively. This increase in potency is even more marked in intact human adipocytes with

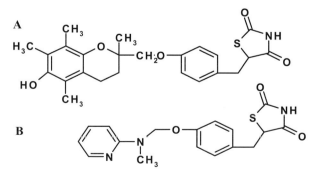

Fig. 8.31 Structures of troglitazone (A) and rosiglitazone (B).

affinities for PPAR-γ of 1050 and 40 nM. Examination of these figures illustrates that troglitazone can be classed as a drug of weak affinity similar to the Na^+ channel blockers.

As a first rule for drug discovery/development programmes it seems prudent to obey the *golden rules* of drug design: Ensure moderate daily dose size by having chosen a viable mechanism and then optimising potency against the target whilst optimising pharmacokinetics. This approach should result in a low dose as exemplified by the anti-diabetic compound troglitazone, a clinical CYP3A4 inducer which has a clinical dose of 200–600 mg, and rosiglitazone a more potent analogue (dose of 2–12 mg), which is devoid of CYP3A4 induction in the clinic. This drive for a low dose also minimises the chances of other toxicities. Polypharmacology is more likely in high dose drugs. For instance the teratogenicity of phenytoin (Fig. 8.29F) has been related to its polypharmacology [48, 49]. The drugs beneficial actions as an anti-convulsant are due to its blockage of Na^+ ion channels (IC_{50} 47 µM). This is a relatively weak activity and hence the high dose nescessary for anti-convulsant activity. Phenytoin is also a blocker of the Ikr channel (HERG ED_{50} 100 µM). Again this is a relatively weak activity, but comparable to the primary pharmacology. Ikr blockers (in laboratory rats) cause bradycardia, arrhythmia and cardiac arrest in the foetus leading to hypoxia, reoxygenation and blood flow alterations [50]. These changes explain the embryonic death, growth retardation, orofacial clefts, distal digital reduction and cardiovascular defects.

8.15
Enzyme Inhibition and Drug Design

All substrates of P450 have the ability to act as competitive inhibitors of CYP450. For many drugs their potency and relatively low dose, plasma concentrations and most importantly liver concentrations, are below the K_m values (typically above 5–50 µM) for their metabolism; therefore, they will not normally cause inhibition drug interactions. Some compounds possess functionality, i.e. their inhibition potential is much greater than their ability to act as a substrate (see below). Some compounds are activated to metastable or stable complexes during metabolism, which become irreversible or slowly reversible inhibitors. These compounds are known as mechanism-based or time-dependent inhibitors. The compounds [51] form stable or quasistable complexes with the enzyme. Binding of the compound is via an oxidised species that binds to the apoprotein, the heme iron or the heme porphyrin. Examples range through antibiotics (erythromycin), anti-cancer agents (tamoxifen), anti-HIV agents (ritonavir), anti-hypertensive agents (mibefradil), steroids (gestodene) and many herbal constituents (bergamolin). The macrolides illustrate the typical activation process to produce the P450 inhibition. The compounds are N-demethylated by P450 to reactive nitrosoalkanes, which form MI-CYP complexes and render the enzyme inactive. Fourteen-membered macrolides such as erythromycin and troleandomycin form these complexes much more readily than 16-membered compounds (azithromycin, spiramycin, etc.).

Lipophilicity is a key factor in binding to cytochrome P450 enzymes (see Section 7.2.3) and it is possible that the SAR for the pharmacological target can be separated from the SAR of the P450. Smith and colleagues [52] give an example where substitution of a sterically hindered heterocycle dramatically alters affinity for CYP1A2, whilst leaving affinity for the target (metabotropic glutamate subtype 5, mglu5) relatively unaffected. Figure 8.32 shows the structure of the thiazole, pyridine and imidazole analogues and their lipophilicity and their relative affinities for mGlu5 and CYP1A2.

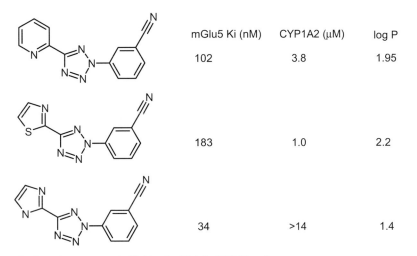

	mGlu5 Ki (nM)	CYP1A2 (µM)	log P
	102	3.8	1.95
	183	1.0	2.2
	34	>14	1.4

Fig. 8.32 Structures and affinities for Mglu5, CYP1A2 and their relationship with lipophilicity in a medicinal chemistry programme to discover metabotropic glutamate subtype 5 receptor antagonists devoid of cytochrome P450 inhibition.

An example of modifications to produce a KCNQ2 potassium channel opener devoid of mechanism-based inhibition is provided by Wu [52]. *(S)*-*N*-[1-(3-morpholin-4-phenyl)ethyl]-3-phenylacrylamide , the original compound, showed excellent oral bioavailability and pharmacological activity (cortical spreading depression preparation for migraine) in animal species but showed time-dependent inhibition of CYP3A4 during *in vitro* testing. Rationalisation of possible metabolism sites and likely reactive quinone intermediates such as that illustrated in Fig. 8.33 allowed the design of the difluoro analogue *(S)*-*N*-[1-(4-fluoro-3-morpholin-4-phenyl)ethyl]-3-(4-fluoro-phenyl)acrylamide. This had comparable pharmacokinetics and pharmacological activity to the original compound, but was devoid of P450 time-dependent inhibition.

Although competitive and rapidly reversible (once concentrations decline), a second group of very potent inhibitors of P450 often include a nitrogen containing heterocycle (pyridine, imidazole or triazole) capable of forming a lone pair ligand interaction with the heme of P450. Such an interaction contributes some 6 kcals

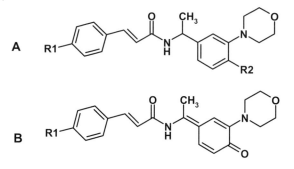

Fig. 8.33 Structures of *(S)-N-[1-(3-morpholin-4-ylphenyl]ethyl]-3-
phenylacrylamide* (A, R1= F, R2 = H) and its difluoro analogue
(R1 = F , R2 = F) designed to block oxidation to a reactive quinone
and resultant P450 inhibition (B).

of binding energy to the interaction (three orders of magnitude increase in
potency). Examples of this class are the azole anti-fungals particularly ketoconazole. Nitrogen-containing heterocyles are essential in many anti-fungal agents as
their target is a P450. The 14-sterol demethylases (CYP51s) catalyze the oxidative
removal of the 14-methyl group of lanosterol to form ergosterol, an important constituent of the cell membrane in fungi, by causing the elimination of 14R methyl
group of lanosterol to give the C14-C15 unsaturated sterol. During the catalytic
cycle, a substrate undergoes three successive mono-oxygenation reactions resulting in formation of 14-hydroxymethyl, 14-carboxaldehyde, and 14-formyl derivatives followed by elimination of formic acid with introduction of a 14, 15 double
bond. The accumulation of 14R-methylated sterols in azole-treated fungal cells
affects membrane structure and functions, resulting in an inhibition of the
growth of fungi. Differential inhibition of this enzyme between pathogenic fungi
and man is the basis for the clinically important activity of these azole anti-fungal
agents. The azole anti-fungal agents in clinical use contain either two or three
nitrogens in the azole ring and are thereby classified as imidazoles (e.g. ketoconazole, miconazole, clotrimazole) or triazoles (e.g. itraconazole, fluconazole, vorico-
nazole), respectively. All are associated with significant drug interactions, needing
high doses (100–400 mg) and relatively high concentrations to achieve efficacy.
Selectivity over the exogenous compound metabolising P450s compared to CYP51
is low.

Another class of drugs also relying on CYP inhibition for efficacy and thus
needing nitrogen containing heterocycles are aromatase inhibitors. Aromatase
(CYP 19) carries out the conversion of androgen to estrogen (i.e. the aromatization
reaction). The first non-steroidal inhibitor was an existing drug: aminoglutethi-
mide. The hypothesis that the AG mode of binding could involve interaction of a
nitrogen atom with the heme iron of CYP19 led to the design of azole-containing
aromatase inhibitors, and from this work emerged drugs such as fadrozole, letro-
zole, vorozole and anastrozole. An excellent example of the importance of target

potency is provided by the later class of aromatase inhibitor. Drug interactions with the azole non-steroidal aromatase inhibitors are much less problematic than with the azole anti-fungal agents. The results of *in vitro* studies show for instance anastrozole can inhibit CYP1A2, 2C9, and 3A4-mediated metabolism at around 10 µM, a concentration predictable from their structure and their relatively low lipophilicity (Fig. 8.34). This potency would not be expected to cause significant interactions in the *in vivo* clinical setting (clinical dose is around 1 mg for these agents): the IC_{50} for inhibition of human placental aromatase activity (15 nM) gives a margin of selectivity of at least 500-fold over inhibition of the drug metabolising CYPs.

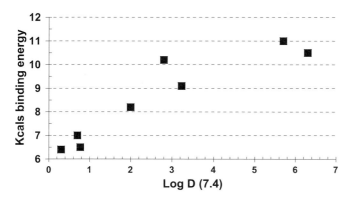

Fig. 8.34 Relationship between lipophilicity and inhibition of CYP3A4 for azole containing 14-sterol de-methylase and aromatase inhibitors.

The use of nitrogen-containing heterocycles is common in medicinal chemistry to increase solubility by replacing an apolar group such as phenyl. Incorporation in a form in which the nitrogen is sterically unhindered will potentially render the compound a potent inhibitor of P450s.

An example where various heterocycles and substitution has been explored to minimise P450 inhibition is provided by Macdonald [53] in the design of dopamine D$_3$ receptor antagonists. The 7-methylsulphonyl-2,3,4,5,-tetrahydro-1*H*-3-benzazepines provide the selected series. Figure 8.35 provides an illustration of a selection of the various five-membered heterocycles tried, all of which gave high selectivity for D$_3$ but varied considerably in their ability to inhibit P450, probably reflecting the steric inhibition of forming the lone pair ligand between the nitrogen atom and the heme.

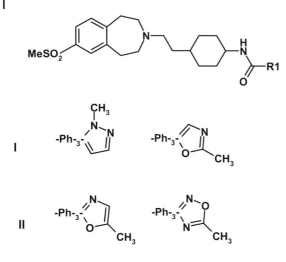

Fig. 8.35 7-Methylsulphonyl-2,3,4,5,-tetrahydro-1*H*-3-benzazepines providing an example of substitution and heterocycle variations in a series of selective D$_3$ antagonists. Hetero-cycles in which R1 is the examples illustrated as I are potent P450 inhibitors. Heterocycles in which R1 is the heterocycles illustrated as II are weak inhibitors.

References

1 Ikeda, K., Oshima, T., Hidaka, H., Takasaka, T. **1997**, *Hearing Res.* 107, 1–8.
2 Kenyon, B., Browne, F., D'Amato, R.J. **1997**, *Exp. Eye Res.* 64, 971–978.
3 Falik, R., Flores, B.T., Shaw, L., Gibson, G.A., Josephson, M.E., Marchlinski, F.E. **1987**, *Amer. J. Med.* 82, 1102–1108.
4 Harris, L., McKenna, W.J., Rowland, E., Holt, D.W., Storey G.C.A., Krikler, D.M. **1983**, *Circulation* 67, 45–51.
5 Smith, D.A., Brown, K., Neale, M.G. **1985–1986**, *Drug Metab. Revs.* 16, 365–388.
6 Nelson, S.D. **1982**, *J. Med. Chem.* 25, 753–761.
7 Hinson, J.A., Roberts, D.W. **1992**, *Ann. Revs. Pharmacol. Toxicol.* 32, 471–510.
8 Cary, R.D., Binnie, C.D. **1996**, *Clin. Pharmacokin.* 30, 403–415.
9 Riley, R.J., Kitteringham, N.R., Park, B.K. **1989**, *Br. J. Clin. Pharmacol.* 28, 482–487.
10 Bennett, G.D., Amore, B.M., Finnell, R.H., Wlodarczyk, B., Kalhorn, T.F., Skiles, G.L., Nelson, S.D., Slattery, J.T. **1996**, *J. Pharmacol. Expl. Ther.* 278, 1237–1242.
11 Tingle, M.D., Jewell, H., Maggs, J.L., O'Neill, P.M., Park, B.K. **1995**, *Biochem. Pharmacol.* 50, 1113–1119.
12 Miyamoto, G., Zahid, N., Uetrecht, J.P. **1997**, *Can. Chem. Res. Toxicol.* 10, 414–419.
13 Spaldin, V., Madden, S., Pool, W.F., Woolf, T.F., Park, B.K. **1994**, *Br. J. Clin. Pharmacol.* 38, 15–22.
14 Ju, C., Uetrecht, J.P. **1998**, *Drug Metab. Dispos.* 26, 676–680.
15 Stonier, P.D. **1992**, *Pharmacoepidemiol. Drug Saf.* 1, 177–185.
16 Roden, D.M. **1995**, Anti-arrhythmic drugs, in *The Pharmacological Basis for Therapeutics*, McGraw-Hill, New York, (pp.) 839–874.

17 Chao, Z., Liu, C., Uetrecht, J.P. **1995**, *J. Pharamacol. Exp. Ther.* 275, 1476–1483.

18 Maggs, J.L., Williams, D., Pirmohamed, M., Park, B.K. **1995**, *J. Pharmacol. Exp. Ther.* 275, 1463–1475.

19 Uetrecht, J., Zahid, N., Tehim, A., Fu, J.M., Rakhit, S. **1997**, *Chemico Biol. Interact.* 104, 117–129.

20 Roberts, P., Kitteringham, N.R., Park, B.K. **1993**, *J. Pharm. Phamacol.* 45, 663–665.

21 Cribb, A.E., Spielberg, S.P. **1990**, *Drug Metab. Dispos.* 18, 784–787.

22 Coleman, M.D. **1995**, *Gen. Pharmacol.* 26, 1461–1467.

23 Treiber, A., Dansette, P.M., Amri, H.E., Girault, J.P., Giderow, D., Mornon, J.-P., Mansy, D. **1997**, *J. Amer. Chem. Soc.* 119, 1565–1571.

24 Mansuy, D. **1997**, *J. Hepatol.* 26(2), 22–25.

25 Wolfe, S.M. **1987**, *New Eng. J. Med.* 316, 1025.

26 Desager, J.P. **1994**, *Clin. Pharmacokin.* 26, 347–355.

27 Liu, Z.C., Uetrecht, J.P. **2000**, *Drug Met. Disp.* 28,726–730.

28 Hepatic monitoring for tenidap **1995**, *Scrip World Pharmaceutical News*, 21, 2073.

29 Durant, G.J., Emmett, J.C., Ganellin, C.R., Miles, P.D., Parsons, M.E., Prain, H.D., White, G.R. **1977**, *J. Med. Chem.* 20, 901–906.

30 Smith, D.A., Johnson, M., Wilkinson, D.J. **1985**, *Xenobiotica* 15, 437–444.

31 Nakadate, M. **1998**, *Toxicol. Lett.* 102–103, 627–629.

32 Begnini, R., Guiliani, A. **1997**, QSAR approaches in mutagenicity and carcinogenecity evaluation, in *Computer-Assisted Lead Finding and Optimization*, Van de Waterbeemd, H., Testa, B., Folkers, G. (eds.), Wiley-VCH, Basel, (pp.) 291–312.

33 Begnini, R., Richard, A.M. **1998**, *Meth.Enzymol.* 14, 264–276.

34 Barratt, M.D. **1998**, *Toxicol. Lett.* 102–103, 617–621.

35 Richard, A.M. **1998**, *Toxicol. Lett.* 102–103, 611–616.

36 Barratt, M.D. **2000**, *Cell Biol. Toxicol.* 16, 1–13.

37 Hall, A.H. **1998**, *Toxicol. Lett.* 102–103, 623–626.

38 Maran, U., Karelson, M., Katritzky, A.R. **1999**, *Quant. Struct. Act. Relat.* 18, 3–10.

39 Vracko, M., Novic, M., Zupan, J. **1999**, *Anal. Chim. Acta* 384, 319–332.

40 Yang, R.S.H., Thomas, R.S., Gustafson, D.L., Campain, J., Benjamin, S.A., Verhaar, H.J.M., Mumtaz, M.M. **1998**, *Environ. Health Perspect. Suppl.* 106, 1385–1393.

41 Cronin, M.T.D. **1998**, *Pharm. Pharmacol. Commun.* 4, 157–163.

42 Olson, H., Betton, G., Stritar, J., Robinsin, D. **1998**, *Toxicol. Lett.* 102–103, 535–538.

43 Sina, J.F. **1998**, *Ann. Rep. Med. Chem.* 33, 283–291.

44 Todd, M.D., Ulrich, R.G. **1999**, *Curr. Opin. Drug Disc. Dev.* 2, 58–68.

45 Nuwaysir, E.F., Bittner, M., Barrett, J.C., Afshari, C.A. **1999**, *Mol. Carcinogen.* 24, 153–159.

46 Kitteringham, N.R., Powell, H., Clement, Y.N., Dodd, C.C., Tettey, J.N.A., Pirmohamed, M., Smith, D.A., McLellan, L.I., Park, B.K. **2000**, *Hepatology* 32, 321–333.

46 Burczynski, M.E., McMillian, M., Ciervo, J., Li, L., Parker, J.B., Dunn, R.T., Hicken, S., Farr, S., Johnson, M.D. **2000**, *Toxicol. Sci.* 58, 399–415.

47 Smith, D.A. **2000**, *Eur. J. Pharm. Sci* 11, 185–189.

48 Salvati, P., Maj, R., Caccia, C., Cervini, M.A., Fornaretto, M.G., Lamberti, E., Pevarello, P., Skeen, G.A., White, H.S., Wolf, H.H., Fararelli, L., Mazzanti, M., Mancinelli, E., Varasi, M., Fariello, R.G. **1999**, *J. Pharm. Exp. Therap.* 288, 1151–1159.

49 Zhou, S., Chan, E., Lim, L.Y., Boelsterli, U.A., Li, S.C., Wang, J., Zhang, Q., Huang, M., Xu, A. **2004**, *Curr. Drug Met.* 5, 415–442.

50 Danielsson, B.R., Skold, A.C., Azarbayjani, F. **2001**, *Curr. Pharm. Des.* 7, 787–802.

51 Smith, N.D., Poon, S.F., Huang, D., Green, M., King, C., Tehrani, L., Roppe, J., Chung, J., Chapman, D.,

Cramer, M., Nicholas, D.P. **2004**, *Bioorganic Med. Chem. Lett.* 14, 5481–5484.

52 Wu, Y.-J., Davis, C.D., Dworetzky, W.C., Fitzpatrick, W.C., Harden, D., He, H., Knox, R.J., Newton, A.E., Philip, T., Polson, C., Sivarao, D.V., Sun, L.-Q., Tertyshnikova, S., Weaver, D., Yeola, S., Zoeckler, M., Sinz, M.W. **2003**, *J. Med. Chem.* 46, 3778–3781.

53 Macdonald, W., Branch, G.J., Hadley, C.K., Johnson, M.S., Nash, C.N., Smith, D.J., Stemp, A.B., Thewlis, G., Vong, K.M., Austin, A.K.K., Jeffrey, N.E., Winborn, P., Boyfield, K.Y., Hagan, I., Middlemiss, J.J., Reavill, D.N., Riley, C., Watson, G.J., Wood, J.M., Parker M., Ashby, R.A. **2003**, *J. Med. Chem.* 46, 4952–4964.

9
Inter-Species Scaling

9.1
Objectives of Inter-Species Scaling

Within the drug discovery setting, a principal aim of pharmacokinetic studies is to be able to estimate the likely pharmacokinetic behaviour of a new chemical entity in man. Only by doing this, is it possible to establish if a realistic dosing regimen may be achieved, in terms of both size and frequency of administration. Ultimately these factors will contribute to whether or not the compound can be used practically in the clinical setting and can thus be a successful drug. It is therefore important that pharmacokinetic data derived from laboratory animals can be extrapolated to man. Such extrapolations are at best only an estimate, but can provide valuable information to guide drug discovery programmes. Understanding the physiological processes which underlie the pharmacokinetic behaviour of a molecule allows a more rational estimation of the profile in man.

When considering the likely pharmacokinetic profile of a novel compound in man, it is important to recognise the variability that may be encountered in the clinical setting. Animal pharmacokinetic studies are generally conducted in inbred animal colonies that tend to show minimal inter-subject variability. The human population contains a diverse genetic mix, without the additional variability introduced by age, disease states, environmental factors and co-medications. Hence any estimate of pharmacokinetic behaviour in man must be tempered by the expected inherent variability. For compounds with high metabolic clearance (e.g. midazolam), inter-individual variability in metabolic clearance can lead to greater than tenfold variation in oral clearance and hence systemic exposure [1].

9.2
Allometric Scaling

Much of the inter-species variation in pharmacokinetic properties can be explained as a consequence of body size (allometry). Consequently it is possible to scale pharmacokinetic parameters to the organism's individual anatomy, biochemistry and/or physiology in such a manner that differences between species

Pharmacokinetics and Metabolism in Drug Design.
Dennis A. Smith, Han van de Waterbeemd, Don K. Walker (Eds.)
Copyright © 2006 WILEY-VCH Verlag GmbH & Co. KGaA, Weinheim
ISBN: 3-527-31368-0

are nullified. Several excellent reviews on allometric scaling are available in the literature [2–7]. Allometric relationships provide an equation of the general form:

$$\text{Pharmacokinetic parameter} = A \cdot BW^a \tag{9.1}$$

Where A is the coefficient (i.e. the intercept on the y-axis of logarithmically transformed data), BW is the body weight and a is the power function (slope of the line).

9.2.1
Volume of Distribution

When considering volume of distribution, an allometric relationship is not surprising as this value will be dependent upon the relative affinity for tissue compared to plasma, and as the make-up of tissues is similar across species the ratio will remain relatively constant. Any species-specific differences in plasma protein binding can be overcome by considering volume of distribution of the unbound drug. Due to its unique dependence amongst pharmacokinetic parameters on body weight, the allometric exponent (a in Eq. 9.1) for volume of distribution is generally around 0.9 to 1.0 [8]. The anti-fungal agent, fluconazole provides an excellent example of the allometric relationship between body weight and volume of distribution [9]. This compound has low plasma protein binding (12%) across species and therefore this does not need to be considered in the comparison. As can be seen from Fig. 9.1, when values for volume of distribution (not weight normalised) are plotted against body weight (BW) on a log–log axis, a linear relationship with high correlation is observed ($r^2 = 0.99$).

The value of 0.98 for the allometric exponent is so close to unity as to make the volume of distribution directly proportional to body weight, i.e. weight normalised volume is an invariant parameter (see Table 9.1). The mean value for the volume of distribution in the eight species is 0.82 ± 0.21 L kg^{-1}.

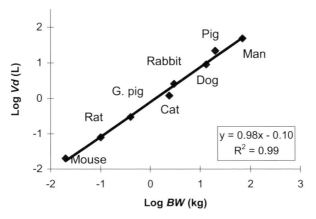

Fig. 9.1 Allometric relationship between body weight and volume of distribution of fluconazole.

Tab. 9.1 Comparison of absolute and weight normalised values for the volume of distribution of fluconazole in various species.

Species	V_d (L)	V_d (L kg^{-1})
Mouse	0.02	1.00
Rat	0.08	0.80
Guinea pig	0.3	0.75
Cat	1.2	0.50
Rabbit	2.6	0.87
Dog	9.1	0.69
Pig	22	1.10
Man	49	0.70

In cases where plasma protein binding varies across the species, allometric scaling should be based upon the volume of distribution of the unbound drug. The considerably lower free fraction (10 to 20-fold) of zamifenacin in human compared to animal plasma results in decreased volume (weight normalised) of the total drug, although the volume of the unbound drug remains constant. This is a major factor in the markedly higher C_{max} (of total drug) after oral dosing in man compared to animal species [10]. This is not always the case for acidic drugs, which are restricted to the blood compartment (typically with a volume of distribution of less than 0.1 L kg^{-1}) as changes in protein binding will not alter the volume of distribution of the total drug.

An extensive retrospective analysis [11] examined various scaling approaches to the prediction of clinical pharmacokinetic parameters. In this analysis the most successful predictions of volume of distribution were achieved by calculating unbound fraction in tissues (f_{ut}) of animals and assuming this would be similar in man. Volume of distribution was then calculated using measured plasma protein binding values and standard values for physiological parameters such as extracellular fluid and plasma volumes. The equation used is as follows:

$$V_{d(human)} = V_p + (f_{u(human)} \cdot V_e) + (f_{b(human)} \cdot R \cdot V_p) + V_r \cdot (f_{u(human)}/f_{ut}) \qquad (9.2)$$

This incorporates volumes of the various fluid compartments, plasma (V_p), extracellular fluid (V_e), and remainder (V_r), in addition to extracellular protein bound drug determined by the ratio of binding proteins in extracellular fluid relative to plasma (R). The predicted volume of distribution calculated by this method had an average fold error of 1.56, with 88% of compounds ($n = 16$) predicted within twofold of the actual value. This method was slightly more reliable than allometric scaling of the volume of distribution of the unbound drug, which provided an average fold error of 1.83, with 77% of compounds ($n = 13$) predicted within two-fold of the actual value. Both methods were significantly better than allometric scaled values without consideration of protein binding differences, which only predicted 53% of compounds ($n = 15$) within twofold of the actual value (average fold error = 2.78).

9.2.2
Clearance

An allometric relationship for clearance is less obvious. However, in many cases the clearance process will be of similar affinity across species. This is particularly so for renal clearance where the processes of filtration and tubular reabsorption are common. In such instances the allometric relationship will be dependent upon organ blood flow. In general, when clearance is expressed in units of volume per unit time per unit of body weight (e.g. mL per min per kg), other mammalian species appear to eliminate drugs more rapidly than man. This is largely a result of the organs of elimination representing a smaller proportion of body weight as the overall size of the mammal increases. For example, the liver of a rat represents approximately 4.5% total body weight, compared to approximately 2.0% for man. The blood flowing to the organ (in this case the liver) is thus reduced when expressed as flow per unit of total body weight from about 100 mL per min per kg in rat to about 25 mL per min per kg in man. When considered another way this means each microlitre of blood in the rat passes though the liver every minute, whereas the equivalent time in man is 2.5 minutes. Thus, everything occurs more rapidly in rat than in man and *physiological time* is shorter (on a chronological scale) the smaller the species. Hence physiological processes that are dependent upon time become disproportionately more rapid in smaller species. This is illustrated by the allometric analysis of creatinine clearance (a measure of glomerular filtration rate), which shows an allometric exponent of 0.69. A similar allometric

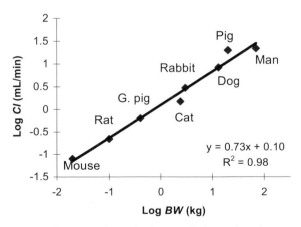

Fig. 9.2 Allometric relationship between body weight and systemic clearance of fluconazole.

exponent is obtained for the clearance of fluconazole (Fig. 9.2), a compound that is almost exclusively renally cleared. Hence, whilst weight normalised clearance may decrease from 4 mL per min per kg in mouse to 0.3 mL per min per kg in man, an allometric relationship is observed across the species with an exponent of 0.73. This value for the exponent is in-keeping with the general observation for small organic molecules where successful predictions are associated with an exponent value of about 0.75 [8]. Thus clearance of fluconazole remains relatively constant with respect to physiological time across the species, as renal clearance remains a constant fraction of glomerular filtration rate (*GFR*) at about 20% [9].

As with the allometric relationship with volume of distribution, fluconazole exhibits only low plasma protein binding and for compounds, which exhibit variation in protein binding across species, allometry should be based upon clearance of the unbound drug. Amongst other renally cleared drugs to show an allometric relationship, the a_1-adrenoceptor antagonist, metazosin, is notable in that the allometric exponent for clearance is 0.28 [12]. Together with the unusual allometric exponent of 0.6 for volume of distribution, this clearly suggests some abnormality in the disposition of this compound which has not yet been explained.

When clearance is dependent upon metabolism, species-specific differences in the enzymes of metabolism can clearly prevent any such allometric relationship. An example of this is the absence of a close homologue of the human CYP2C9 enzyme in the dog, hence its inability to hydroxylate drugs such as tolbutamide and tienilic acid [13]. This said, many compounds cleared by metabolism do exhibit allometric relationships (e.g. *N*-nitrosodimethylamine) [14]. In an extensive analysis of the allometric relationship between clearance in rat and man for 54 extensively cleared drugs, the mean allometric exponent value was 0.66 [15]. This analysis also confirmed the improved correlation when unbound plasma clearance was considered.

9.3
Species Scaling: Adjusting for Maximum Life Span Potential

Allometric scaling of clearance is least successful for metabolically cleared drugs with low extraction. This is perhaps hardly surprising, as these compounds will be most sensitive to the subtle differences in the affinities of species-specific homologues of the enzymes of metabolism. In these cases the clearance in man is generally lower than would be predicted by straightforward allometry. By including a factor that reflects the reduced rate of maturation in man, these differences can be corrected. Such factors have included maximum life span potential (MLP) and brain weight [16].

Compounds which are substrates for mixed function oxidase enzymes, including P450s, tend to show lower than expected clearance in man based upon the simple allometric scaling incorporating body weight alone. This may be correlated with the enhanced longevity of man compared to animals, since the faster the pace of life, the shorter it is. Hence slowing the metabolic rate, including that of the mixed function oxidases, allows the MLP to be extended. This reflects a major evolutionary advantage of man over other animal species. Therefore incorporation of MLP into the allometric extrapolation provides a more accurate assessment of physiological time than body weight alone. One additional potential advantage of reduced activity of the mixed function oxidases is decreased activation of procarcinogens and decreased free radical formation, hence prolonging life span.

The consideration of clearance in units of volume per maximum life span potential, instead of the traditional volume per weight, provides an allometric relationship for drugs such as antipyrine and phenytoin [17]. Both of these drugs are essentially low-clearance compounds, cleared by P450 metabolism. Ultimately, the successful utility of such factors may be purely serendipitous as they simply exploit unique features of man as a species.

9.4
Species Scaling: Incorporating Differences in Metabolic Clearance

An alternative approach to relying simply upon allometric approaches for metabolically cleared compounds is to take into consideration the relative stability *in vitro*. Clearance by P450 enzymes observed in hepatic microsomes from different species provides a measure of the relative intrinsic clearance in the different species. Using the equation for the well-stirred model:

$$Cl_s = \frac{Cl_i \cdot Q}{(Cl_i + Q)} \tag{9.3}$$

The equation can be solved for intrinsic clearance (Cl_i) based upon systemic clearance (Cl_s) obtained after IV administration and hepatic blood flow (Q) in the test species. Intrinsic clearance in man can then be estimated based upon relative *in vitro* microsomal stability and the equation solved to provide an estimate for human systemic clearance. Hence this approach combines allometry (by considering differences in organ blood flow) and species-specific differences in metabolic clearance.

The incorporation of *in vitro* metabolism data into allometric scaling of compounds cleared by hepatic metabolism has been extensively evaluated [18] and shown to accurately predict human clearance. In this review it is suggested that the utility of such methods are most appropriately applied in drug candidate selection, to confirm early estimates and to support early clinical studies.

The inclusion of relative metabolic stability in animal and human hepatocytes into allometric scaling for ten metabolically cleared compounds has been detailed [19]. In this study, the correction for species differences in metabolic rate resulted in extrapolated human clearance values within twofold of those observed. In contrast, extrapolations based on simple allometry or incorporating a correction for brain weight gave up to tenfold errors on the extrapolated values. Again in these approaches to scaling, differences in plasma protein binding can be incorporated using the equation:

$$Cl_i = Cl_{iu} \times f_u \qquad\qquad\qquad (9.4)$$

Where f_u is the fraction unbound in plasma of the relevant species. Extrapolation based on unbound drug clearance is generally the approach of choice for estimating metabolic clearance in man prior to progressing a compound into clinical trials [20].

A comparison of various inter-species scaling methods was conducted for the endothelin antagonist, bosentan [21]. This compound is eliminated mainly through metabolism. Simple, direct allometric scaling based on five animal species provided a relatively poor correlation coefficient (r^2) of 0.53. Whilst the r^2 value was greatly improved (0.90) by correcting for brain weight, this gave a relatively poor prediction of human clearance of 44 mL min⁻¹ versus an actual value of 140 mL min⁻¹. The best r^2 value (0.98) was obtained by correcting for rates of metabolism in hepatocytes from the various species and this also provided a relatively good prediction of human clearance at 100 mL min⁻¹. Whilst the correlation coefficient was inferior when incorporating metabolic stability in liver microsomes (0.73) instead of hepatocytes, this also provided a good estimate of human clearance at 126 mL min⁻¹. In this example no account was taken of plasma protein binding differences between species.

9.5
Inter-Species Scaling for Clearance by Hepatic Uptake

When transporter proteins are involved in the rate-determining step of compound clearance, there is clearly the potential for species differences to exist which are not related to allometry. Given the large (and growing) number of transporter proteins implicated in the removal of drugs from the systemic circulation (see Chapter 5), there exists the possibility for divergent substrate specificity in the various laboratory animal species and man.

Organic anions have frequently been implicated as substrates for transporters in the sinusoidal membrane of the liver. This was illustrated for a series of TxRAs,

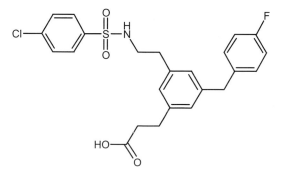

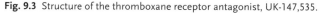

Fig. 9.3 Structure of the thromboxane receptor antagonist, UK-147,535.

where hepatic uptake was identified as the rate-determining step in the clearance process [22]. A representative compound from this series, UK-147,535 (Fig. 9.3), was progressed to clinical trials [23]. It is thus possible to contrast clearance of this compound between a number of species including man (Fig. 9.4).

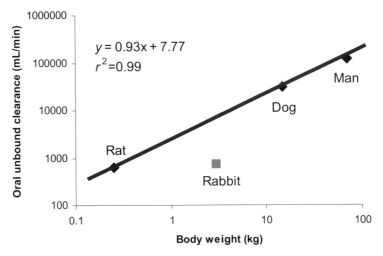

Fig. 9.4 Allometric relationship for clearance of UK-147,535 in various species.

As observed in Fig. 9.4 the intrinsic clearance (as represented by oral unbound clearance Cl_{ou}) of UK-147,535 shows an allometric relationship between rat, dog and man. This would indicate that the transporter protein involved is conserved across these species and has similar affinity. However, marked reduction in clearance in the rabbit suggests the absence, or marked alteration, of the responsible protein in the hepatic sinusoidal membrane of this species. This finding may explain the common observation of reduced biliary excretion of acidic compounds in rabbits compared to other species [24, 25].

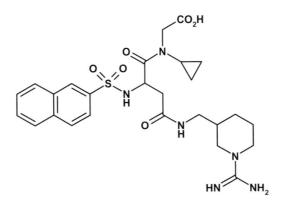

Fig. 9.5 Structure of the thrombin inhibitor, napsagatran.

It remains to be established if other transporter proteins for other drug classes (e.g. cations) are conserved between species. Active transport processes are believed to be involved in the renal and hepatic clearance of the zwitterionic thrombin inhibitor, napsagatran (Fig. 9.5). Allometric scaling based on pharmacokinetic data from rat, rabbit, monkey and dog overestimated total clearance, non-renal clearance and volume of distribution in man by three, seven and twofold, respectively. As napsagatran is not metabolised *in vitro* or *in vivo*, this would suggest that species differences in the transport proteins involved in the clearance of napsagatran, especially the protein responsible for hepatic uptake across the sinusoidal membrane, compromise the kinetic extrapolations from animals to man. Notably, amongst the individual species investigated, the monkey was most predictive of human clearance and volume of distribution [26].

9.6
Elimination Half-Life

The relationship between elimination half-life ($t_{1/2}$) and body weight across species results in poor correlation, most probably because of the hybrid nature of this parameter [27]. A better approach may be to estimate volume of distribution and clearance by the most appropriate method and then estimate half-life indirectly from the relationship:

$$t_{1/2} = \frac{0.693 \times V_d}{Cl_s} \qquad (9.5)$$

9.7
Scaling to Pharmacological Effect

The ultimate aim of all pharmacokinetic scaling is to predict the potential pharmacological utility of a novel compound in clinical use. This requires linking the projected plasma concentration profile derived from the predicted pharmacokinetic parameters to projected efficacy concentrations or indeed safety thresholds when considering potential adverse events. For compounds where free drug concentrations are considered an appropriate measure of the drug concentration available to exert a pharmacological effect (e.g. receptors and ion channels with extracellular access), this can be readily assessed by use of projected free drug exposure as illustrated in Fig. 9.6 [28]. With regard to the value of such pharmacokinetic predictions in relation to drug safety, application of a safety threshold of 30-fold between therapeutically active concentrations and those eliciting prolongation of the QT interval has been proposed for the assessment of risk to the form of ventricular tachycardia known as *torsades de pointes* [29].

The pharmacological target concentrations may be refined depending on the available preclinical data and may include the inclusion of pharmacokinetic/phar-

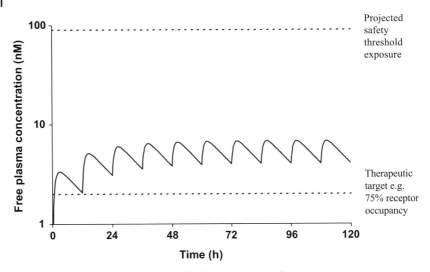

Fig. 9.6 Modeled pharmacokinetic profile of a novel chemical entity with consideration of free drug exposure relative to projected efficacy levels (based on receptor occupancy) and safety threshold (based on level at which QT prolongation is anticipated).

macodynamic (PK/PD) data from animal studies if available. However, the modeling may also be relatively crude, in order to assess the relative impact of changes in potency and pharmacokinetics on the overall predicted dosing requirements within a drug discovery programme.

An example of this is provided within a drug discovery programme to identify a potent and M3 selective antimuscarinic agent (this series is also discussed in Chapter 7). A number of potential candidates were assessed with variations in pharmacological and pharmacokinetic properties. The lead compound in this programme (compound I, Fig. 9.7), possessed excellent potency (pA_2 = 8.8) but exhibited high clearance in pre-clinical species and projected high clearance in man, based upon extrapolations of clinical pharmacokinetics, using animal and *in vitro* information, with an estimated unbound intrinsic clearance in man of around 1300 mL per min per kg. Crude estimates of the required exposure to exhibit a pharmacological effect based upon maintaining concentrations averaging three times the pA_2 value for 24 hours allow estimation of the required dose using the equation:

$$\text{Dose} = Cl_{iu} \cdot \text{AUC} \qquad (9.6)$$

This provided an estimated dose of 300 mg per day for compound I without any consideration at this time for required dosing frequency, although high clearance and short elimination half-life would indicate a short duration of action. In order to improve upon this profile a number of more polar analogues of compound I were investigated in order to reduce the intrinsic clearance of the compounds.

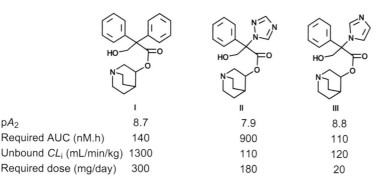

	I	II	III
pA_2	8.7	7.9	8.8
Required AUC (nM.h)	140	900	110
Unbound CL_i (mL/min/kg)	1300	110	120
Required dose (mg/day)	300	180	20

Fig. 9.7 Structure of M3 selective antimuscarinic compounds with estimates of required systemic exposure (free AUC), based on potency and required dose based on the required exposure and predictions of human unbound intrinsic clearance derived from animal and *in vitro* pharmacokinetic data.

The triazole analogue (compound II, Fig. 9.7) exhibited markedly reduced clearance, leading to a longer half-life in animals and *in vitro* preparations, but reduced potency (pA_2 = 7.9), and led to a similar dose requirement estimation of 180 mg per day. Only in the imidazole analogue (compound III, Fig. 9.7) where potency was retained and clearance reduced did this significantly impact on the projected dose, which was reduced to 20 mg per day. In addition the reduced clearance of this compound indicated that this compound had greater potential to provide efficacious drug concentrations with twice daily dose administration.

9.8
Single Animal Scaling

In a drug discovery environment rapid decisions must be made based on the prediction of human *in vivo* pharmacokinetics (PK). This necessitates a minimum amount of animal *in vivo* data. At early stages bulk drug is at a minimum so work is practically confined to the rodent. Caldwell and colleagues [30] have investigated the accuracy of the *in vivo* correlation between rat and human for the prediction of the total systemic clearance (CL), the volume of distribution at steady state (V_{ss}), and the half-life ($t_{1/2}$) using simple allometric scaling techniques. They demonstrated that (using a large diverse set of drugs) a fixed exponent allometric scaling approach could be used to predict human *in vivo* PK parameters CL, V_{ss} and $t_{1/2}$ solely from rat *in vivo* PK data with acceptable accuracy. The best allometric scaling relationships were $CL_{Human} = 40\ CL_{Rat}$ (L hour^{-1}), $V_{ssHuman} = 200\ V_{ssRat}$ (L), and $t_{1/2Human} = 4\ t_{1/2\ Rat}$ (hour). The average fold error for human CL predictions for $N = 176$ drugs was 2.25 with 79% of the drugs having a fold error less than three. The average fold error for human V_{ss} predictions for $N = 144$ drugs was 1.85 with 84% of the drugs having a fold error less than three. The average fold error for human $t_{1/2}$ predictions for $N - 145$ drugs was 2.05 with 76% of the drugs having a fold error less than three. When corrected for body weight differences (human 70 kg, rat 0.25 kg) the major scaling consideration is that man has a clearance approximately sevenfold lower than rat (see Section 9.2.2). Single species approaches provide a pragmatic alternative to total reliance on *in vitro* approaches. In some ways they mimic an earlier and successful pharmacology screening paradigm of oral studies in rodents from which many gastrointestinal and cardiovascular drugs were discovered.

References

1 Wandel, C., Bocker, R.H., Bohrer, H., deVries, J.X., Hofmann, W., Walter, K., Klingeist, B., Neff, S., Ding, R., Walter-Sack, I., Martin, E. **1998**, *Drug Metab. Dispos.* 26, 110–114.

2 Boxenbaum, H. **1981**, *J. Pharmacokin. Biopharm.* 10, 201–227.

3 Boxenbaum, H., D'Souza, R. **1988**, *NATO ASI Ser. Ser. A*, vol. 145.

4 Hayton, W.L. **1989**, *Health Physics* 57, 159–164.

5 Paxton, J.W. **1995**, *Clin. Exp. Pharm. Physiol.* 22, 851–854.

6 Mahmood, I., Balian, J.D. **1996**, *Life Sciences* 59, 579–585.

7 Ritschel, W.A., Vachharajani, N.N., Johnson, R.D., Hussain, A.S. **1992**, *Comp. Biochem. Physiol.* 103C, 249–253.

8 Mordenti, J. **1986**, *J. Pharm. Sci.* 75, 1028–1040.

9 Jezequel, S.G. **1994**, *J. Pharm. Pharmacol.* 46, 196–199.

10 Beaumont, K.C., Causey, A.G., Coates, P.E., Smith, D.A. **1996**, *Xenobiotica* 26, 459–471.

11 Obach, R.S., Baxter, J.G., Liston, T.E., Silber, M., Jones, B.C., MacIntyre, F., Rance, D.J., Wastall, P. **1997**, *J. Pharm. Exp. Ther.* 283, 48–58.

12 Lapka, R., Rejholec, V., Sechser, T., Peterkova, M., Smid, M. **1989**, *Biopharm. Drug Dispos.* 10, 581–589.

13 Smith, D.A. **1991**, *Drug Metab. Rev.* 23, 355–373.

14 Gombar, C.T., Harrington, G.W., Pylypiw, H.M., Anderson, L.M., Palmer, A.E., Rice, J.M., Magee, P.N., Burak, E.S. **1990**, *Cancer Res.* 50, 4366–4370.

15 Chou, W.L., Robbie, G., Chung, S.M., Wu, T.-C., Ma, C. **1998**, *Pharm. Res.* 15, 1474–1479.

16 Ings, R.M.J. **1990**, *Xenobiotica* 20, 1201–1231.

17 Campbell, D.B., Ings, R.M.J. **1988**, *Human Toxicol.* 7, 469–479.

18 Lave, T., Coassolo, P., Reigner, B. **1999**, *Clin. Pharmacokinet.* 36, 211–231.

19 Lave, T., Dupin, S., Schmitt, C., Chou, R.C., Jaeck, D., Coassolo, P. **1997**, *J. Pharm. Sci.* 86, 584–590.

20 Smith, D.A., Jones, B.C., Walker, D.K. **1996**, *Med. Res. Rev.* 16, 243–266.

21 Lave, T., Coassolo, P., Ubeaud, G., Bradndt, R., Schmitt, C., Dupin, S., Jaeck, D., Chou, R.C. **1996**, *Pharm. Res.* 13, 97–101.

22 Gardner, I.B., Walker, D.K., Lennard, M.S., Smith, D.A., Tucker, G.T. **1995**, *Xenobiotica* 25, 185–197.

23 Dack, K.N., Dickinson, R.P., Long, C.J., Steele, J. **1998**, *Bioorg. Med. Chem. Lett.* 8, 2061–2066.

24 Simons, P.J., Cockshott, I.D., Douglas, E.J., Gordon, E.A., Knott, S., Ruane, R.J. **1991**, *Xenobiotica* 21, 1243–1256.

25 Illing, H.P.A., Fromson, J.M. **1978**, *Drug Metab. Dispos.* 6, 510–517.

26 Lave, T., Portmann, R., Schenker, G., Gianni, A., Guenzi, A., Girometta, M.-A., Schmitt, M. **1999**, *J. Pharm. Pharmacol.* 51, 85–91.

27 Mahmood, I. **1998**, *J. Pharm. Pharmacol.* 50, 493–499.

28 Walker, D.K. **2004**, *Br. J. Clin. Pharmacol.* 58, 601–608.

29 Webster, R., Leishman, D., Walker, D. **2002**, *Curr. Opin. Drug Discov. Devel.* 5, 116–126.

30 Caldwell, G.W., Masucci, J.A., Yan, Z., Hageman, W. **2004**, *Eur. J. Drug Met. Pharmacokinet.* 29, 133–143.

10
High(er) Throughput ADME Studies

10.1
The High-Throughput Screening (HTS) Trend

New approaches to medicinal chemistry such as parallel synthesis and combinatorial chemistry strategies [1], and refinement of high-throughput screening in biology place drug discovery at a crossroads. Will traditional rational medicinal chemistry continue as the cornerstone of how we discover drugs or will shear numbers of compounds be the winning formula. High compound numbers are essential, whatever the eventual scenario to ensure that early lead matter is available. The size of compound files of the future, millions of compounds, means informatics and automation are key ingredients for a successful drug discovery organisation [2]. How much drug metabolism needs to adapt is part of the question. Clearly many of the *in vitro* approaches can be automated and drive efficiencies. These systems are equally adaptable to screening a file or providing fast turnaround on newly synthesised products of a rational discovery programme. Both approaches are being pursued. This chapter discusses the place of ADME screens and describes some of the recent developments to give insight into how medicinal chemistry in the not too far future may benefit.

10.2
Drug Metabolism and Discovery Screening Sequences

The development of higher-throughput approaches in ADME studies is driven by the advances in high-speed chemistry and pharmacological screening [3], a view of the future that many more compounds would need to be screened and the availability of the technology. Departments of drug metabolism and pharmacokinetics in the pharmaceutical industry are organising themselves for the rapid evaluation of large numbers of compounds [4–9]. Higher throughput can move a screening approach up the traditional sequence, provide more comprehensive data on a single compound, or just screen more compounds or even files. The pre-ADME days of discovery had screening sequences based on an *in vitro* functional response often followed by an oral rodent pharmacodynamic model. The

Pharmacokinetics and Metabolism in Drug Design.
Dennis A. Smith, Han van de Waterbeemd, Don K. Walker (Eds.)
Copyright © 2006 WILEY-VCH Verlag GmbH & Co. KGaA, Weinheim
ISBN: 3-527-31368-0

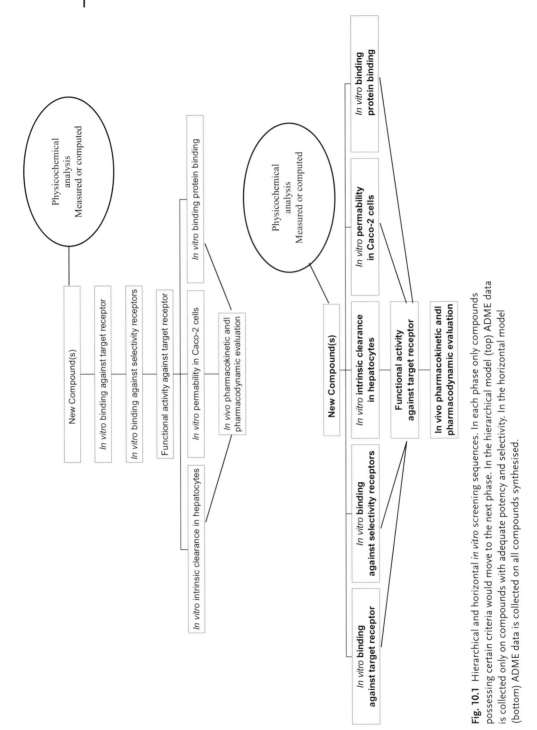

Fig. 10.1 Hierarchical and horizontal *in vitro* screening sequences. In each phase only compounds possessing certain criteria would move to the next phase. In the hierarchical model (top) ADME data is collected only on compounds with adequate potency and selectivity. In the horizontal model (bottom) ADME data is collected on all compounds synthesised.

advent of ADME, cloned receptors, etc., has led to the hierarchical sequence shown in Fig. 10.1. Higher throughput could allow a parallel process, which collects large amounts of *in vitro* pharmacology and ADME data as the primary stage.

The hierarchical model is closest to the traditional approach and meets the needs of a focussed, disciplined approach, where molecules are drug-like, with a real possibility of passing some of the ADME criteria. The horizontal model is optimum for looking for exceptions to drug-like property rules and can build SAR streams much more rapidly, therefore, allowing for very comprehensive real-time SAR of the type normally reserved for retrospective analysis. These two models indicate a divergence of how the data are handled. The hierarchical model means that full data are available on a few compounds, can be manipulated on a spreadsheet and are within the brainpower of a medicinal chemist. This relates to the data being unimportant and the learned elements are retained to drive the process. The horizontal model could result in more than 5000 data points to collate as SAR. This immediately requires computational systems and complex analysis to process and optimise. Some progress has been made in methods used in early ADME evaluation [6] with *in silico* and higher-throughput physicochemical methods being linked to appropriate *in vitro* models [7]. The following sections give an inventory of some of these approaches.

10.3
Physicochemistry

The importance of physicochemistry to drug disposition and ADME is summarised in tabular form as Table 10.1.

Tab. 10.1 Physicochemical properties and the relationship to key disposition processes. Number of ticks indicates relative importance and the arrow indicates how an increase in the physicochemical property affects the ADME property, e.g. dissolution is decreased by increasing lipophilicity.

	Lipo-philicity	Molecular size	Hydrogen bonding	Ionisation	Melting point, crystal packing
Dissolution	✓✓✓ ↓			✓✓	✓✓✓ ↓
Membrane permeation, lipoidal	✓✓✓ ↑	✓✓	✓✓	✓	
Membrane permeation, aqueous		✓✓✓ ↓			
Non-specific binding to proteins and phospholipids	✓✓✓ ↑			✓✓✓	
Carrier transport					
Metabolism	✓✓✓ ↑			✓	
Renal clearance	✓✓✓ ↓				

10.3.1
Solubility

Solubility is a key parameter for dissolution of compounds following oral admin-istration (Section 3.1). The process depends on the surface area of the dissolving solid and the solubility of the drug at the surface of the dissolving solid. Solubility is inversely proportional to the number and type of lipophilic functions within the molecule and the tightness of the crystal packing of the molecule. Rapid, robust methods reliant on turbidimetry to measure solubility have been developed [10, 11], which can handle large numbers of compounds. Since ionisation can also govern solubility, approaches for the rapid measurement of pK_a values of spar-ingly soluble drug compounds have also been developed [12]. Ideally only soluble compounds would be synthesised in a discovery programme, which is where pre-dictive solubility methods using neural networks [13, 14] would be such an advan-tage.

10.3.2
Lipophilicity

Lipophilicity is the key physicochemical parameter linking membrane permeabil-ity, and hence drug absorption and distribution with route of clearance (metabolic or renal). Measured or calculated lipophilicity of a compound is readily amenable to automation. Many of these calculation approaches rely on fragment values, but a simple method based on molecular size to calculate log P values has been dem-onstrated to be extremely versatile [15]. A combination of measured and fragmen-tal approaches allow prediction of extremely accurate new compound properties. For actual measurement rather than prediction, investigations in using alterna-tives to octanol/water partitioning include applications of immobilised artificial membranes (IAM) [16] and liposome/water partitioning [17, 18]. The IAM meth-od offers speed of measurement as an advantage over the classical octanol/water system. Liposome binding may possibly be transferred to a higher-throughput sys-tem and could provide a volume of distribution screen when linked with other properties. Hydrogen-bonding capacity of a drug solute is now recognised as an important constituent of the concept of lipophilicity. Initially Δlog P, the differ-ence between octanol/water and alkane/water partitioning, was used as a measure for solute H-bonding, but this technique is limited by the poor solubility of many compounds in the alkane phase. Computational approaches to this range from simple heteroatom counts (O and N), division into acceptors and donors, and more sophisticated measures such as free energy factors (used in *Hybot*) and polar surface area (*PSA*).

10.4
Absorption/Permeability

When a compound is crossing a membrane by purely passive diffusion, a reasonable permeability estimate can be made using single molecular properties such as log D or hydrogen bonding (see Chapters 1 and 3). Currently *in vitro* methods such as Caco-2 monolayers are widely used to make absorption estimates (see Chapter 3). The trend is to move to 24 and to 96-well plates, but this is possibly the limit for this screen in its current form. New technologies need to be explored. Artificial membranes such as PAMPA have been suggested for high-throughput permeability assessment [19–23]. However, besides the purely physicochemical component contributing to membrane transport, many compounds are affected by biological events including the influence of transporters and metabolism. Many drugs appear to be substrates for transporter proteins, which either promotes or is detrimental to permeability. Currently no theoretical SAR basis exists to account for these effects. Ultimately, the fastest method is to make absorption estimates *in silico* (see Chapter 3) [24, 25]. Learning of all above approaches needs to be put into those systems before these can be reliable and truly predictive.

10.5
Pharmacokinetics

Important progress in terms of higher throughput in ADME/PK work was realised recently by wider use of liquid chromatography/mass spectrometry (LC/MS), which has now become a standard analytical tool [26]. Flow NMR spectroscopy has become a routine method to resolve and identify mixtures of compounds and has found applications in drug metabolism and toxicology studies [27].

Mixture dosing (*n-in-one* dosing, or cocktail dosing, or cassette dosing) has been explored as a means to get higher throughput [28–30]. Efficient groupings may consist of 10 to 25 compounds. In order to avoid potential interactions the dose should be kept as low as possible. Another approach is the analysis of pooled plasma samples and the use of an abbreviated standard curve per compound [31]. From an estimated AUC a ranking of compounds offers early PK information.

A rapid spectrofluorimetric technique for determining drug-serum protein binding in high-throughput mode has been described [32].

P-glycoprotein-mediated efflux is a potential source of peculiarities in drug pharmacokinetics, such as non-linearity. This includes dose-dependent absorption, drug–drug interactions, intestinal secretion and limited access to the brain. Assays are in development to quantify the interaction between transporters and drugs. One of the first are a 96-well plate assay for P-gp binding [33, 34] and a MDR1 ATPase test [35].

10.6
Metabolism and Inhibition

As outlined in Sections 6.2 and 6.3 the balance between renal clearance and metabolism can be predicted by physicochemical considerations [36].

Much of metabolism can be broadly predicted from similar considerations, however whilst lipophilicity is a key factor in metabolic stability, the influence of functionality is also very high. The metabolic stability of compounds can be assayed in a high-throughput or semi-high-throughput screening system using recombinant enzymes, human liver microsomes or human hepatocytes. The use of mass spectrometry, in particular triple quadrupole instruments provide universal detectors for many of these *in vitro* systems, and separation systems are continually evolving to allow more and more direct introduction of sample [37]. The choice of reagent governs the breadth of metabolic processes examined. The recombinant enzyme [38–40], normally CYP3A4, obviously only studies reactions performed by that enzyme. However some 75% of all drugs are cleared predominantly by the enzyme, so screening against this enzyme will provide useful SAR. Microsomal systems with the appropriate co-factors provide a comprehensive screening reagent, although some oxidation systems are absent (soluble) such as aldehyde oxidase, and some conjugation systems such as sulpho-transferase. In most cases screening is run using the microsomes fortified with NADPH (via a regenerating system) to study P450 metabolism (and flavin mono-oxygenases). Broad screening for metabolic stability is best accomplished with hepatocytes, which provide a system containing all the enzyme systems: oxidative, conjugative and hydrolytic. In terms of ease of use, the hierarchy is reversed as hepatocyte systems are difficult to obtain, difficult to cryopreserve, and generally show limited linearity against cell concentration. This means in terms of measuring stability hepatocytes have a lower dynamic range. Human systems also suffer from the variability of the donor(s) and even when pooled into fairly large batches show differences in metabolic rate across batches. Screening results are normally percentage remaining or described by disappearance half-life. This is convertible into intrinsic clearance using appropriate scaling, a parameter which has a pharmacokinetic significance (see Section 2.3).

The potential for compounds to inhibit the major human cytochrome P450 isoenzymes is now routinely assessed during the discovery stage as a high-throughput screen. Normally recombinant enzymes are used together with relatively nonselective fluorescent probe substrates [41], the selectivity being gained by use of the individual isoforms. These screens tend to use a single substrate concentration (around 24–50 μM) and look for percentage inhibition of the reaction against control. Depending on the design of the screen all types of inhibitors are examined. Incubations are conducted with and without a 15 minute pre-incubation. This allows both the rapidly reversible competitive inhibitors and the time-dependent mechanism-based inhibitors (see Section 8.14) to be identified. The latter class of inhibitor is recognised by an increasing inhibition of the reaction with time. More detailed IC_{50} can be obtained by examining the reaction over a broader concentration range. Human liver microsomes are sometimes used with much lower throughput (often in later development stages). Here selective drug substrates are employed. IC_{50} values are initially obtained for compounds against CYPs 1A2, 2C9, 2C19, 2D6, 2E1 and 3A4. Respective substrates for these isoenzymes, phenacetin, diclofenac, S-mephenytoin, bufuralol, chlorzoxazone and testosterone are incubated at a concentration equal to their K_m value with the test compound (concentration range generally 0.01 to 1000 µM). For comparison purposes positive control inhibitors (e.g. ketoconazole, CYP3A4) for the isoforms are routinely incorporated in the study. If the IC_{50} value (which approximates to $2 \times K_i$) is below 50 µM for any isoform, then K_i values are determined for that reaction

10.7
The Concept of ADME Space

Clearly there is a need for optimal pharmacokinetics in development candidates to maximise the chances of these compounds becoming marketed drugs. Optimum pharmacokinetics are often not ideal pharmacokinetics since the optimisation of a drug molecule includes potency, selectivity, etc. To understand the optimisation process, the various components of activity that make up a drug can be

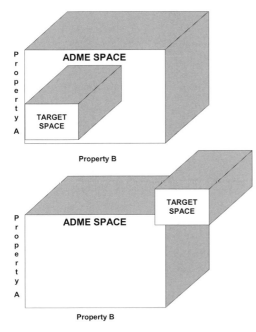

Fig. 10.2 The concept of target and ADME space. Properties could be physicochemical such as number of H-bonding functions, sum of the number of nitrogen and oxygen atoms (property A), and molecular weight (property B). The top example shows a target within ADME space the bottom figure one on the limits of ADME space.

viewed as occupying an area of space bounded by acceptable properties. A molecule must exist in overlapping target space, selectivity space and ADME space to be a drug. This is illustrated in Fig. 10.2, as the top example.

The properties A and B could refer to physicochemical properties such as number H-bonding functions and lipophilicity (or molecular weight), respectively. Targets such as adrenoceptors illustrate this since the basic requirements for agonism or antagonism are satisfied with a minimum of these properties. The properties also have direct correlation with ADME properties such as membrane permeability (absorption) and metabolic stability. The rule of five, which was described in Section 3.3 and was the result of analysis of marketed drugs, is a simple model for ADME space. The space is bounded by the molecular weight and its constituents (C, N or O). As molecular weight moves towards 500, if the constituents are largely carbon, then lipophilicity becomes very high, adversely affecting dissolution and metabolic clearance, whilst incorporation of N and O in high numbers offsets this but adversely effects membrane transfer due to the size of the water sheaf limiting adsorption and maximising the effect of transporters.

Failure of these spaces to overlap means the target is *undruggable* by small molecules. New techniques continue to rapidly change the drug discovery environment. Genomics inputs new targets, similarly high-throughput screening technologies have been followed by high-speed chemical synthesis. The use of these can accelerate lead identification by rapid screening of large compound libraries. Moreover, the technology also replaces or supports the traditional labour and time intensive process of turning chemical leads into development candidates by rational synthesis. Traditional agonists and antagonists of targets such as aminergic 7TMs occupy a target space surrounded by ADME and selectivity space as described above. As we move away from these targets to others, such as non-aminergic 7TMs (those in which the natural ligand is a peptide, etc.) the overlap of target and ADME space is often severely restricted (see Section 3.3 for medicinal chemistry approaches to move into ADME space with ligands to these types of receptors). Optimum molecules may become very much the exception and are actually a compromise. Finding the overlap between ADME space and target space and exploring within this requires a combination of traditional medicinal chemistry rationale design aligned to the use of high-speed synthetic and screening techniques.

The role of ADME space is illustrated when MW (molecular weight), $\log P$ (lipophilicity) and $\log S_w$ (intrinsic water solubility) drugs were compared [42] for HTS leads, compounds in the medicinal chemistry phase (lead development) and compounds in development (phases I, II ,III and launched). The lead structures show the lowest median with respect to MW (smaller) and $\log P$ (less hydrophobic), and the highest median with respect to $\log S_w$ (more solubility). By contrast, over 50% of the lead development compounds had $MW > 425$, $\log P > 4.25$ and $\log S_w < -4.75$, indicating that the active compounds are larger, more hydrophobic and less soluble than the lead material. This is a natural trend to gain affinity (optimise target space) potentially moving out of ADME space. The development compounds show a progressive constraint to reduce MW and $\log P$, and to increase log S_w, across phase I, II, III and launched drugs. The filtering out in development of compounds partly reflects the constraints of ADME and the likelihood of good ADME properties.

10.8
Computational Approaches in PK and Metabolism

A number of approaches are available or under development to predict metabolism, including expert systems such as MetabolExpert (Compudrug), Meteor (Lhasa), MetaFore [42] and the databases Metabolite (MDL) and Metabolism (Synopsys) [43]. Ultimately such programs may be linked to computer-aided toxicity prediction based on quantitative structure–toxicity relationships and expert systems for toxicity evaluation such as DEREK (Lhasa) (see also Chapter 8) [44].

QSAR and neural network approaches in combination with physiologically-based pharmacokinetic (PBPK) modelling hold promises to become a powerful tool in drug discovery [45]. Below we briefly discuss some of these studies.

10.8.1
QSPR and QSMR

As a possible alternative to *in vitro* metabolism studies, QSAR and molecular modelling may play an increasing role. Quantitative structure–pharmacokinetic relationships (QSPR) have been studied for nearly three decades [42, 45–52]. These are often based on classical QSAR approaches based on multiple linear regression. In its most simple form, the relationship between PK properties and lipophilicity has been discussed by various workers in the field [36, 49, 50].

Similarly, quantitative structure–metabolism relationships (QSMR) have been studied [42]. QSAR tools, such as pattern recognition analysis, have been used to predict phase II conjugation of substituted benzoic acids in the rat [53].

10.8.2
PK Predictions Using QSAR and Neural Networks

Neural networks are a relatively new tool in data modelling in the field of pharmacokinetics [54–56]. Using this approach, non-linear relationships to predicted properties are better taken into account than by multiple linear regression [45]. Human hepatic drug clearance was best predicted from human hepatocyte data, followed by rat hepatocyte data, while in the studied data set animal *in vivo* data did not significantly contribute to the predictions [56].

10.8.3
Is *In Silico* Meeting Medicinal Chemistry Needs in ADME Prediction?

Stouch and co-workers [57] have suggested why the *in silico* revolution has not happened despite the promise of the above methods and others described in the literature. Their paper (*In Silico ADME/Tox: Why Models Fail*) describes several case examples which actually apply very often generically.

Data quality. To gain a large enough data set, literature data is employed. Such data will span many laboratories and will have been collected under varying experimental protocols and conditions. The data set therefore is actually worthless. Even in a single laboratory data collected over time will often show variation. An example would be human microsomal or hepatocyte clearance. It is common practice to pool these reagents to try to lower variations; individual human samples showing huge variation in certain enzymes. For example, the major human CYP (CYP3A4) shows a 20 to 25-fold variation across a series of human livers. Despite pooling, substantial variation can be seen between pooled batches. Even with the appropriate positive controls it is difficult to build a large data set from such screens. The commonly used Caco-2 cell line system shows variation in result due to cell passage numbers, culture time, type of support and medium. Hou and colleagues [58], in describing the correlation of Caco-2 permeation with simple molecular properties, highlight the variation in laboratory data. Their training data set the P_{eff} for mannitol, often used as a quality standard, showed in tenfold variation across referenced studies (–6.75 cf. – 5.49). Their approach in *curating* the published data indicates the difficulty in literature-derived training sets. The authors also point out, the somewhat more surprising ranges encountered in measured hydrophobicity descriptors such as log $D_{7.4}$. They note again a near tenfold variation in values for compounds as exemplified by atenolol (–1.29 cf. –2.14).

Other aspects can also be added in that certain data are very hard to obtain. Whilst human bioavailability data are readily available these data are a composite of fraction of the drug absorbed, gut first-pass metabolism and liver first-pass metabolism. To obtain human absorption per se as a true permeability value and relate that to Caco-2 or replace such screens is thus highly problematic. Likewise most of the data on blood-brain penetration are derived from animal experiments comparing whole blood or plasma with total brain. Such data are only of limited use compared to CSF or ECF concentration data.

- Compound space. Almost invariably any model will fail. No matter how many compounds are employed to build a data set, chemists will innovate and make structures dissimilar to those used to build the model. In the example from Stouch [57], the model was based on 800 marketed drugs. These compounds showed only a very low similarity (less than 0.3 on a scale from zero to one) to those being investigated as putative drugs.
- Accuracy around critical decision points. Many screening cascades have a cut-off point to either test the compound further or

to seek an alternative compound. These cut-off points are based on project wisdom and sometimes pragmatism. Many models can show a general trend, but fail to have any predictive value around a go/no go value. Stouch's example [57] is a decision of CYP2D6 inhibition. Although the model was 90% predictive, the go/no go point was 10 µM. Here the model predicted correctly 60% of the time and falsely 40% of the time.

In a similar vein, a description of a solubility model gives a description where even if accuracy had been achieved the dynamic range did not address the key areas of interest. In this model the lowest limit was 1 µM for poorly soluble compounds. With potent molecules solubility below this value may be adequate. Moreover, progress in improving solubility from very low levels could not be predicted.

Although somewhat gloomy the paper does highlight that both the *in silico* models and the way they are used need to be harmonised to make a full impact on medicinal chemistry.

10.8.4
Physiologically-Based Pharmacokinetic (PBPK) Modelling

There are several approaches to pharmacokinetic modelling. These include empirical, compartmental, clearance-based and physiological models. In the latter, full physiological models blood flow to and from all major organs and tissues in the body are considered. Such models can be used to study concentration–time profiles in the individual organs, e.g. in the plasma [59–62]. Further progress in this area may result in better PK predictions in humans [63]. Ideally such models would be able to start with basic screening data and incorporate new data in a holistic manner. Table 10.1 indicates how lipophilicity is important in many of the processes we describe in this book, and just simple measurement of it or calculation allows some predictions to be made (e.g. drug clearance, see Section 5.4). Refinement by data from permeability and metabolism screens would increase the accuracy of prediction. Larger data sets would be obtained for compounds of specific interest. It is hoped that such systems are developed and introduced to aid drug discovery.

10.9
Outlook

Ultimately rapid methods are needed to obtain data adequate at each stage of drug discovery. At the candidate selection level, the extrapolation from animals to man, through the integration of pharmacokinetics and pharmacodynamics (PK/PD), becomes crucial for success [64, 65]. Such HT methods are currently being implemented and further developed in the pharmaceutical and biotech industry [66]. *In silico* approaches, including prediction, modelling and simulation, are being evaluated and eventually will be integrated in the screening sequence to become the *in combo* approach to drug discovery [67].

References

1 Antel, J. **1999**, *Curr. Opin. Drug Discov. Dev.* 2, 224–233.
2 Calvert, S., Stewart, F.P., Swarna, K., Wiserman, J.S. **1999**, *Curr. Opin. Drug Disc. Dev.* 2, 234–238.
3 Tarbit, M.H., Berman, J. **1998**, *Curr. Opin. Chem. Biol.* 2, 411–416.
4 Rodrigues, A.D. **1997**, *Pharm. Res.* 14, 1504–1510.
5 Rodrigues, A.D. **1998**, *Med. Chem. Revs.* 8, 422–433.
6 Smith, D.A. **1998**, *Biomed. Health Res.* 25, 137–143.
7 Eddershaw, P.J., Beresford, A.P., Bayliss, M.K. **2000**, *Drug Discov. Today* 5, 409–414.
8 White, R.E. **2000**, *Ann. Rev. Pharmacol. Toxicol.* 40, 133–157.
9 Smith, D.A., Van de Waterbeemd, H. **1999**, *Curr.Opin.Chem.Biol.* 3, 373–378.
10 Avdeef, A. **1998**, *Pharm. Pharmacol. Commun.* 4, 165–178.
11 Lipinski, C.A., Lombardo, F., Dominy, B.W., Feeney, P.J. **1997**, *Adv. Drug Del. Revs.* 23, 3–25.
12 Allan, R.I., Box, K.J., Coomer, J.E.A., Peake, C., Tam, K.Y. **1998**, *J. Pharm. Biomed. Anal.* 17, 699–710.
13 Huuskonen, J., Salo, M., Taskinen, J. **1998**, *J. Chem. Inform. Comput. Sci.* 38, 450–456.
14 Huuskonen, J., Salo, M., Taskinen, J. **1997**, *J. Pharm. Sci.* 86, 450–454.
15 Buchwald, P., Bodor, N. **1998**, *Curr. Med. Chem.* 5, 353–380.
16 Ong, S., Liu, H., Pidgeon, C. **1996**, *J. Chromatogr. A.* 728, 113–128.
17 Ottiger, C., Wunderli-Allenspach, H. **1997**, *Eur. J. Pharm. Sci.* 5, 223–231.
18 Balon, K., Riebesehl, B.U., Muller, B.W. **1999**, *J. Pharm. Sci.* 88, 802–806.
19 Kansy, M., Kratzat, K., Parrilla, I., Senner, F., Wagner, B. **2000**, in *Molecular Modelling and Prediction of Bioreactivity*, Gundertofte, K., Jorgensen, F. (eds.), Plenum, New York, (pp.) 237–243.
20 Kansy, M., Senner, F., Gubernator, K. **1998**, *J. Med. Chem.* 41, 1007–1010.
21 Kansy, M. **2001**, in *Pharmacokinetic Optimization in Drug Research: Biological, Physicochemical and Computational Strategies*, Testa, B., Van de Waterbeemd, H., Folkers, G., Guy, R. (eds.), Wiley-HCA, Zurich.
22 Avdeef, A. **2001**, in *Pharmacokinetic Optimization in Drug Research: Biological, Physicochemical and Computational Strategies*, Testa, B., Van de Waterbeemd, H., Folkers, G., Guy, R. (eds.), Wiley-HCA, Zurich.
23 Faller, B., Wohnsland, F. **2001**, in *Pharmacokinetic Optimization in Drug Research: Biological, Physicochemical and Computational Strategies*, Testa, B., Van de Waterbeemd, H., Folkers, G., Guy, R. (eds.), Wiley-HCA, Zurich.
24 Van de Waterbeemd, H. **2001**, in *Pharmacokinetic Optimization in Drug Research: Biological, Physicochemical and Computational Strategies*, Testa, B., Van de Waterbeemd, H., Folkers, G., Guy, R. (eds.), Wiley-HCA, Zurich.
25 Krämer, S.D. **1999**, *Pharm. Sci. Tech. Today* 2, 373–380.
26 Unger, S.E. **1999**, *Ann. Rep. Med. Chem.* 34, 307–318.
27 Stockman, B.J. **2000**, *Curr. Opin. Drug Disc. Dev.* 3, 269–274.
28 Adkinson, K.K., Halm, K.A., Shaffer, J.E., Drewry, D., Sinhababu, A.K., Berman, J. **1998**, in *Integration of Pharmaceutical Discovery and Development: Case Histories*, Borchardt, R.T., Freidinger, R.M., Sawyer, T.K., Smith, P.L. (eds.), Plenum Press, New York, (pp.) 423–443.
29 Shaffer, J.E., Adkinson, K.K., Halm, K., Hedeen, K., Berman, J. **1999**, *J. Pharm. Sci.* 88, 313–318.
30 Bayliss, M.K., Frick, L.W. **1999**, *Curr. Opin. Drug Disc. Dev.* 2, 20–25.
31 Cox, K.A., Dunn-Meynell, K., Korfmacher, W.A., Broske, L., Nomeir, A.A.,

Lin, C.C., Cayen, M.N., Barr, W.H. **1999**, *Drug Discov. Today* 4, 232–237.

32 Parikh, H.H., McElwain, K., Balasubramanian, V., Leung, W., Wong, D., Morris, M.E., Ramanathan, M. **2000**, *Pharm. Res.* 17, 632–637.

33 Döppenschmitt, S., Langguth, P., Regardh, C.G., Andersson, T.B., Hilgendorf, C., Spahn-Langguth, H. **1999**, *J. Pharmacol. Exp. Ther.* 288, 348–357.

34 Döppenschmitt, S., Spahn-Langguth, H., Regardh, C.G., Langguth, P. **1998**, *Pharm. Res.* 15, 1001–1006.

35 Sarkadi, B., Price, E.M., Boucher, R.C., Germann, U.A., Scarborough, G.A. **1992**, *J. Biol. Chem.* 267, 4854–4858.

36 Smith, D.A., Jones, B.C., Walker, D.K. **1996**, *Med. Res. Rev.* 3, 243–266.

37 Van Breemen, R.B., Nikolic, D., Bolton, J.L. **1998**, *Drug Metab. Dispos.* 26, 85–90.

38 Crespi, C.L. **1999**, *Curr. Opin. Drug Discov.* 2, 15–19.

39 Crespi, C.L., Miller, V.P., Penman, B.W. **1998**, *Med. Chem. Res.* 8, 457–471.

40 Crespi, C.L., Miller, V.P., Penman, B.W. **1997**, *Anal. Biochem.* 248, 188–190.

41 Palamanda, J.R., Favreau, L., Lin, C., Nomeir, A.A. **1998**, *Drug Discov. Today* 3, 466–470.

42 Oprea, T. **2000**, *Molecular Diversity* 5, 199–208.

42 Testa, B., Cruciani, G. **2001**, in *Pharmacokinetic Optimization in Drug Research: Biological, Physicochemical and Computational Strategies*, Testa, B., Van de Waterbeemd, H., Folkers, G., Guy, R. (eds.), Wiley-HCA, Zurich.

43 Ehrhardt, P. W. (ed.) **1999**, *Drug Metabolim Databases and High-Throughput Testing During Drug Design and Development*, IUPAC, Blackwell Science, Malden, MA.

44 Cronin, M.T.D. **1998**, *Pharm. Pharmacol. Commun.* 4, 157–163.

45 Van der Graaf, P.H., Nilsson, J., Van Schaick, E.A., Danhof, M. **1999**, *J. Pharm. Sci.* 86, 306–312.

46 Hansch, C. **1972**, *Drug Metab. Revs.* 1, 1–14.

47 Seydel, J.K., Schaper, K.J. **1982**, *Pharmac. Ther.* 15, 131–182.

48 Mayer, J.M., Van de Waterbeemd, H. **1985**, *Environm. Health Perspect.* 61, 295–306.

49 Toon, S., Rowland, M. **1983**, *J. Pharmacol. Exp. Ther.* 225, 752–763.

50 Walther, B., Vis, P., Taylor, A. **1996**, in *Lipophilicity in Drug Action and Toxicology*, Pliska, V., Testa, B., Van de Waterbeemd, H. (eds.), VCH, Weinheim, (pp.) 253–261.

51 Seydel, J.K., Trettin, D., Cordes, H.P., Wassermann, O., Malyusz, M. **1980**, *J. Med. Chem.* 23, 607–613.

52 Hinderling, P.H., Schmidlin, O., Seydel, J.K. **1984**, *J. Pharmacokin. Biopharm.* 12, 263–287.

53 Cupid, B.C., Holmes, E., Wilson, I.D., Lindon, J.C., Nicholson, J.K. **1999**, *Xenobiotica* 29, 27–42.

54 Hussain, A.S., Johnson, R.D., Vachharajani, N.N., Ritschel, W.A. **1993**, *Pharm. Res.* 10, 466–469.

55 Brier, M.E., Zurada, J.M., Aronoff, G.R. **1995**, *Pharm. Res.* 12, 406–412.

56 Schneider, G., Coassolo, P., Lavé, T. **1999**, *J. Med. Chem.* 42, 5072–5076.

57 Stouch, T.R., Kenyon, J.R., Johnson, S.R., Chen, X.Q., Doweyko, A., Li, Y. **2003**, *J. Comput. Aided Mol. Des.* 17, 83–92.

58 Hou, T.J., Zhang, W., Quiao, X.B., Xu, X.J. **2004**, *J. Chem. Info. Sci.* 44, 1585–1600.

59 Yoshikawa, Y., Sone, H., Yoshikawa, H., Takada, K. **1999**, *Yakubutsu Dotai* 14, 22–31.

60 Iwatsubo, T., Hirota, N., Ooie, T., Suzuki, H., Sugiyama, Y. **1996**, *Biopharm. Drug Dispos.* 17, 273–310.

61 Kawai, R., Mathew, D., Tanaka, C., Rowland, M. **1998**, *J. Pharmacol. Exp. Ther.* 287, 457–468.

62 Poulin, P., Theil, F.P. **2000**, *J. Pharm. Sci.* 89 16–35.

63 Norris, D.A., Leesman, G.D., Sinko, P.J., Grass, G.M. **2000**, *J. Contr. Rel.* 65, 55–62.

64 Campbell, D.B. **1996**, *Ann. N.Y. Acad. Sci.* 801, 116–135.

65 Campbell, D.B. **1998**, *Biomed. Health Res.* 25, 144–158.

66 Van de Waterbeemd, H., Kohl, C. (eds.), **2004**, *Drug Disc Today: Technol.* 1, 337–463.

67 Dickens, M., Van de Waterbeemd, H. **2004**, *BioSilico* 2, 38–45.

Index

Pharmacokinetics and Metabolism in Drug Design.
Dennis A. Smith, Han van de Waterbeemd, Don K. Walker (Eds.)
Copyright © 2006 WILEY-VCH Verlag GmbH & Co. KGaA, Weinheim
ISBN: 3-527-31368-0